STATISTICS
for Healthcare Professionals

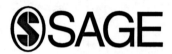

Ian Scott and Debbie Mazhindu

STATISTICS
for Healthcare Professionals

An Introduction

SECOND EDITION

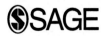

Los Angeles | London | New Delhi
Singapore | Washington DC

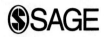

Los Angeles | London | New Delhi
Singapore | Washington DC

SAGE Publications Ltd
1 Oliver's Yard
55 City Road
London EC1Y 1SP

SAGE Publications Inc.
2455 Teller Road
Thousand Oaks, California 91320

SAGE Publications India Pvt Ltd
B 1/I 1 Mohan Cooperative Industrial Area
Mathura Road
New Delhi 110 044

SAGE Publications Asia-Pacific Pte Ltd
3 Church Street
#10-04 Samsung Hub
Singapore 049483

Editor: Alison Poyner
Associate editor: Emma Milman
Production editor: Katie Forsythe
Copyeditor: Neil Dowden
Proofreader: Mary Dalton
Indexer: David Rudeforth
Marketing manager: Tamara Navaratnam
Cover design: Wendy Scott
Typeset by: C&M Digitals (P) Ltd, Chennai, India

Library of Congress Control Number: 2013948136

British Library Cataloguing in Publication data

A catalogue record for this book is available from
the British Library

ISBN 978-1-4462-0893-9
ISBN 978-1-4462-0892-2 (pbk)

Contents

About the Authors

Ian Scott is Associated Dean for Student Experience in the Faculty of Health and Life Science at Oxford Brookes University. He has worked in higher education for over 20 years and in 2011 was awarded a National Teaching Fellowship. Ian's main research area is learning in non-classroom environments. He has published in areas such as experiential learning in professional education, the recognition of prior learning and the role of fieldwork in environmental education. Ian's love of statistics developed through his first degree which is in Applied Biology. Ian lives with his family in Great Malvern, UK and in his spare time enjoys sailing and cycling.

Debbie Mazhindu is Reader in Clinical Practice Innovation in the Faculty of Society and Health, Buckinghamshire New University (BNU) and Imperial Healthcare NHS Trust. Debbie has over 24 years teaching experience and has worked in senior management and strategic levels within six different universities in the UK and abroad. Debbie is a qualified Nurse (Adult), Nurse Tutor and Registered Practice Educator (NMC), and has over 16 years clinical experience in: Intensive Therapy and Coronary Care, Accident & Emergency, Medical and Surgical and Care of Older People.

Acknowledgements

We would like to acknowledge all those students we have worked with that have helped us to develop our approach to teaching the use of statistics to Health professionals. We would also like to thank the publisher's editorial team who, as always, have done so much.

The author and publisher would like to thank Kathie Moore for her contribution to the initial work on the first edition of this text.

Additional Online Material

Additional online material focuses on use of well know computer programmes that are currently used to analyse statistics. The material guides users in how to undertake, the various statistical tests described in the textbook using statistical software. It will give access to the data sets of the hypothetical studies outlined in Chapter 5. Through using the resources you will become more practiced and adept at analysing data with statistics.

 Visit www.sagepub.co.uk/scott2e for access to the following materials which accompany the book:

Guide to using Microsoft Excel
Guide to using SPSS
Datasets

1

Statistics for health care research

Areas of learning covered in this chapter

How can you use this book and use statistics to enhance practice?
What is evidence-based practice (EBP)?
How are statistics used to enhance evidence-based health care?
How can statistics help you to evaluate professional knowledge and professional values as the evidence base for practice?

Scope of the book

This book aims to expand health care students' and professionals' knowledge and understanding of statistics within health care practice. We hope that through reading and using this book you will be encouraged to evaluate statistical analysis as a technique and its relationship to evidence-based practice, and develop a practical understanding of basic statistics. There are many different approaches to investigating questions in health care practice. We deal with quantitative approaches to investigating problems in health care, which require an understanding of some of the rules and principles of statistics. Understanding research in health care requires appreciating both qualitative and quantitative approaches to analysing data. Students of health care professions, both medical and non-medical, can expect to encounter a range of research approaches, which use particular statistical techniques to derive answers to particular patient problems. To this end, health care practice involves understanding of a range of research techniques within health-related subjects, including the use of statistics.

> **Glossary** When you see a term in **bold** you may want to look it up in the glossary of terms at the end of the book. This will explain terms used and help you to remember key words.

For many students and practitioners of health care, statistics is a subject that can often appear incomprehensible, daunting and, worse still, far removed from the real issues and problems encountered when caring for people. Within the book we try to demystify some of the more commonly used statistical tests and help readers understand the language of research that uses statistics, which both novice and advanced researchers find very off-putting to read. Undertaking the exercises within and at the end of each chapter will encourage you to think critically and reflectively about the research that you encounter, both in terms of the statistical process and the dynamic health care context in which studies are executed. The book can be used as a basis for taught courses on statistics at both pre-registration and post-registration level and as a reference guide for those using statistics in health care settings. The book is an introduction and aims to take you from novice to advanced beginner. Statistics is a vast subject which many people find difficult. We hope to make the learning process easier, but we can't promise an effort-free process.

The book is divided into twenty chapters. Each contains explanations of its terms and use for reference. A glossary has been provided and every time you encounter a word in **bold** print you can look up a short definition in the glossary. At the end of each chapter you will find questions and exercises. Using these exercises will allow you to practise, become more proficient and develop your understanding.

The book takes a 'how to' approach, which explains how specific statistical tests can be performed. We have included details of how to calculate many of the statistics by hand, because doing at least some of the statistics by hand will help you to get a feel for the processes. As the statistical techniques become more advanced, readers are directed towards suitable computer packages and other literature. Understanding statistics can sometimes be difficult for students of health care, as statistics often appear far removed from immediacy of patient problems. Examples of statistical techniques commonly used will be explored and the results of a hypothetical questionnaire on sexual health and a clinical trial are used to encourage you to practise and explore statistics. We encourage you to try calculating statistics by hand, at least at first as this will help you to develop a feel for what is going on. Computers with statistical packages are now more readily available in some health care settings, particularly in the more industrialized parts of the world. As tests become more advanced and you feel more confident, do try to use the statistical computer packages that are available. (A short guide to using SPSS and Excel can be found at www.sagepub.co.uk/scott2e.)

The use of clinical and community-based studies will form a central thread to allow data analysis to be explored from the perspective of differing subject areas. As well as analysing data from the studies provided we encourage you to analyse your own data, collected in response to some sample questions.

We encourage you to think critically about data analysis and research design and how appropriate research design impacts upon evidence-based practice, because an understanding of statistics is essential if the numerous reports and documents issued within the health industries are to be scrutinized and considered in a critical manner.

Box 1.1   Reflective exercise

Take a few moments to think about the decisions made in health care today.

- How do we make decisions about what is the best care for patients and clients?
- How do you make decisions about what is best for you?
- How do you feel about making decisions that may affect another person's life?
- How do you feel about people's health?
- How do you feel about circumstances which may affect a person's ability to: give birth, father or mother children, recover from cancer, cope with devastating trauma, cope with loss or grief, help someone integrate back into society after mental illness?

How do we as health care providers analyse such problems and then come to reach decisions that have an impact on many people's lives? The answers to these questions lie in the basis we use for our professional knowledge, the power we have to implement changes in practice and what constitutes our evidence base for our practice.

After reading this book, we hope that your skills of critical analysis will have become more refined. We anticipate that you will have a better understanding of the process of research and the use of statistics and all that is involved in getting answers to problems. We hope that you will be able to understand the importance of carefully reading and reviewing research reports in order to come to conclusions about their relevance to your area of practice. It is also hoped that you will begin to feel comfortable talking the language of quantitative research, which can assist you when presenting a case for changing or improving an area of practice.

The use of statistics in health care research

There has been an increase in the development of research-based and evidence-based practice (EBP) in health care over the last two decades. For students undertaking professional health care education and those practising as professionals in health care, understanding the statistical terms used in research is of paramount importance when evaluating research studies.

One of the key aims of this text is to enable the development of a greater understanding of the process and practice of using statistics in order to find answers to complex health problems. After the initial preparation to practise health care, qualified practitioners are charged with a duty to care for patients and clients in the best manner possible. This means: taking account of patients' and clients' family life and their involvement with others, the knowledge and skills attributed to practice, medical orders and the role of the allied health professions (AHPs). Understanding statistical terms and analysis helps practitioners to make sense of the many research studies that underpin EBP, takes account of professional values as service providers to the public and enables practitioners to undertake studies themselves.

What are the goals of health care research?

The primary goal of health care research is to aid patient and client care by developing a scientifically based body of knowledge, which can be used to help us with decision making, to develop new practice and promote the professional role. The degree to which a body of people such as health care professionals can be judged as professional resides to a large extent on the body of specialist knowledge that they can draw on for practice. Developing a specialist knowledge base by a process of scientific enquiry can aid the professional standing of a professional health care provider. The ultimate aim of health care providers is the delivery of safe, effective care for patients and clients. This is an essential prerequisite in all health care professionals' codes of conduct.

   Understanding statistics is just one way of ensuring that professional practice is based on the best available evidence to date by which to treat and help the wider community. Health care research shares many of the qualities of practice interventions, as they are both practical and intellectual activities, which have a defined language to learn. Good practice and good research do not spring from *ad hoc* or sloppy practice. Health care practice and health care research both use processes which when applied rigorously can improve patient care. Health care practice that is ritualized, not research-based and not assessed, not planned and (more importantly) not evaluated to see if it makes a difference to patient care can kill people, as it leads to unsafe practice. Evidence of this is to be found in the various catalogues of disciplinary hearings concerned with the safe conduct of health care providers of all disciplines.

Box 1.2   Professional values

Take a look at this set of values, which are common to most health care professions; how do you think a knowledge of statistical analysis could help you to maintain these values?

- To practise within the various codes of conduct, which regulate your chosen health care discipline.
- Be aware of cause and effect of health and ill health.
- Track progression and regression of health states and disease.
- Serve society by implementing the best practice based on available evidence.
- Teach new generations of health care professionals by using up-to-date research findings.
- To be self-governing and self-regulating in order to protect and serve the public.

Randomized control trials (RCTs)

Currently in health care practice, the 'gold standard' type of research is the randomized control trial (RCT) but even this kind of research has its critics and is not immune from accusations concerning its truthfulness and the way RCTs are conducted. For example, there are disagreements about how many RCTs should be undertaken before the outcomes can be used as evidence, how big the samples are to be legitimized as '**representative**' and how 'international' a range of samples are before data is acceptable as 'significant'. An RCT is a highly specialized research undertaking as usually the patients are carefully selected prior to randomization; usually they are younger and healthier than the people who will actually be taking the drug, and the people in the sample selected will only usually have one thing wrong with them and only be taking that one drug. Conversely, people in the 'real world' will be older and very likely have two or three conditions for which they are also taking five or more drugs making comparisons difficult if not impossible. RCTs do, however, remain the 'gold standard' form of research in health care.

The fact remains that research, from whichever perspective, that is not rigorous, systematic, ethical and well designed can have devastating effects on people's lives. The thalidomide drug research is a case in point. Maynard (2003) suggested that medication errors occurring in health care in the United States kill twice the number of people per year than those who died in the terrorist attack on the World Trade Center on 11 September 2001. The prevalence of Methicillin-resistant *Staphylococcus aureus* (MRSA) and other resistant microbes causes great concern across the globe. In France, four times more antibiotics are consumed *per capita* than among Dutch patients, with higher levels of antibiotic resistance as a result (ibid.). Understanding statistics in health care research, then, is every professional health care provider's business.

Professional knowledge and evidence-based practice

Currently, many hospitals in the UK gather systematic and routine statistical data (often called metrics) from patient care settings, in order to determine the effectiveness of the service provided and to determine the prevalence and incidence of iatrogenesis[1] such as: the number and incidence/prevalence of patient falls, health care induced infections (especially catheter acquired urinary tract infection), pressure ulcers, patient complaints, drug administration errors or cases of inadequate nutrition. It is essential that health care providers are able to interpret and act appropriately upon these data.

The demand of EBP today for implementing practice based upon statistical evidence is still problematic (Raleigh and Foot 2010). The difficulties can be attributed to a large extent to the lack of understanding of statistics, lack of understanding about effective training of data gatherers, sample size, sampling techniques, timeframes and methods of data collection and, lastly, the lack of engagement of health care providers in the process of change (Maynard 2003). Instituting change in health care relies on an understanding of statistics. Understanding the language of statistics gives all health care providers a common language despite the differences between the professions. The difficult question remains of gaining consensus in deciding what exactly constitutes evidence.

---

[1] An iatrogenic disorder is a condition that is caused by health: treatment, care, personnel or through exposure to the environment of a health care facility.

Box 1.3

Take ten minutes to write down possible sources of evidence you have seen routinely gathered in the clinical area you are working in; this could relate to, for example, staffing levels, sickness absence, patient complaints, bed occupancy, staff vacancies, incidences of MRSA, admissions, deaths and discharges.

- Can you identify when and at what time this data is collected?
- Does the time this data is collected (e.g. midnight) represent a fair and accurate representation of incidence/prevalence of the evidence?

If we examine the credibility of evidence-based practice (EBP) in health care through exploration of its philosophical origins, there are several key features that emerge as important considerations. First, we need to evaluate critically the declared purposes and strengths of what exactly constitutes the evidence base for practice in health care. Second, we require an analysis of the implicit reasons for implementation of EBP. Third, we require a critical discussion of the strengths and limitations of EBP within the context of modern health care. An example of this is the data collection for metrics used in many UK hospitals. Following the publication of the recent Francis (2013) report which identified cases of poor quality care and lack of compassion that have subsequently become the focus of much media attention in the UK, now more than ever health care workers and their leaders need to identify the way statistical evidence and measurement can be used to best effect (Royal College of Nursing (RCN) 2009) and to demonstrate good patient outcomes (NHS Outcomes Framework 2012/2013). Measuring the quality of care is central to providing in good patient care (NHS IC 2010) that is more transparent, accountable and focused on improvement (Maben et al. 2012). The brief outline below attempts to articulate in terms of numerical measures 'quality of nursing care', illustrating some of the issues surrounding the wider use of EBP but also how understanding what phenomena to measure and how they can be measured is so important for health care practitioners and managers of health care services.

A report by Maben et al. (2012), for example, draws together information about a wide range of UK initiatives and international developments in the measurement of nursing quality and describes:

- current knowledge and issues about use of nursing metrics;
- types of nursing metrics that are currently being used in the English National Health Service (NHS);
- national and international trends in measurement of nursing;
- the feasibility of a national set of key indicators of high-quality nursing;
- design and implementation of an infrastructure that enables national consistency and benchmarking between organizations.

It remains unclear, however, the extent to which all of these variables are sensitive to variations in nursing quality as there are numerous other contextual variables that impact upon the quality of patient care, which can be regarded as wider structural indicators and therefore beyond the realm of nursing to effect any measurable difference (ibid.), and these normally fall to the responsibility of senior management, such as:

- workforce, e.g. staffing levels, skill mix, sickness absence, recruitment and retention;
- staff experiences, e.g. perception of the practice environment, ongoing education training and continuing professional and personal development (CPPD);
- systems, e.g. admissions, discharge, handover, medically led health care administration.

The collection and use of statistical data in care quality metrics, if developed and used in the right way, has the potential to support and improve all areas of care delivered through the NHS in England (Mabon et al. 2012). For example, indicators and metrics included in *Imperial College Healthcare NHS Trust Quality Improvement Framework* (Gage et al. 2012) are:

1. Nurse sensitive outcome indicators: care bundle compliance (falls prevention, pressure ulcer prevention, food and nutrition, pain and failure to rescue), incidence and prevalence data relating to falls, pressure ulcers and catheter-acquired urinary tract infections.
2. Infection prevention and control: hand hygiene compliance, invasive devices care bundle compliance, cleaning scores, incidence data for trust acquired MRSA and *C. diff* cases, MRSA screening rates.
3. Workforce: band and agency usage, sickness, vacancy and appraisal rates.
4. Patient experience: commissioning for quality and innovation scores, complaints.

Whilst in the UK many NHS trusts[2] are measuring some or all of these indicators in a structured way at a local level (see North West Transparency Project UK), including the use of 'quality dashboards' (Royal College of Nursing (RCN) 2011), there is still considerable overlap between approaches to quality measurement but, as yet, lack of standardization of key quality indicators (Maben et al. 2012). This means that in the UK many current systems of measurement do not permit effective benchmarking between organizations and at the ward or unit level (ibid.). Whilst there appears to be some degree of standardization around specific nursing quality indicators for patient safety, including measures for falls and pressure sores (the NHS Safety Thermometer, and through the North West Transparency Project), there is a dearth of good risk adjustment for measures such as falls and pressure ulcers to ensure valid comparisons between organizations within the UK (ibid.). Very few UK metrics systems appear to have achieved the advanced metrics systems represented by the United States and Canada (ibid.).

It is questionable whether EPB is flawed, a borrowed or unique concept, but whichever the view, it is better than doing nothing to ensure better safer patient care. What is clear is the need for staff undertaking EBP to understand the basics of statistics in order to understand metrics. Whatever considerations and issues are raised with EBP, there can be no doubt about the impact of statistics upon the prevailing views of professional health care practice. The implications of ensuing debate on statistical concepts for health care providers are numerous and have

---

[2] Publicly owned organizations that provide and organize health care in the UK under the NHS are known as NHS trusts.

significant implications for the future of the professions, because these range from immediate curriculum development and delivery of professional practice in health care education and training to a multi-professional and multicultural perspective, including the role and preparation of educators, clinicians and students. The **quantitative paradigm** has had a massive impact on the knowledge base for the practice of health care professionals. Some authors (Colyer and Kamath 1999) maintain that, philosophically, EBP is fundamentally utilitarian. If that is the case, an understanding of statistics is essential for EBP.

Having read this chapter and completed the exercises, you should be familiar with the following ideas and concepts:

- using this book to develop your understanding of statistics;
- evidence-based practice;
- the relationship between quantitative research and evidence-based practice;
- how quantitative research contributes to the development of professional knowledge and professional values;
- the importance of statistics in health care practice.

EXERCISES

1. When considering introducing change to your practice, what type of evidence do you require to support that change?
2. Consider the last time change was introduced to your practice. What evidence was it based on? What role did you play in the decision? Did the change have a statistical basis?

2

The statistical approach: when should it be applied?

Areas of learning covered in this chapter

- What are the major concepts in statistical analysis?
- What types of studies use statistical analyses?
- Where do statistics fit within the research framework?

In our first chapter we discussed how an understanding of statistics is essential if professionals are to engage with the development of professional knowledge and practice. But what are statistics? Why use the statistical approach and when should it be applied? How do we know if the right test has been used when reading and evaluating research?

What are statistics?

Statistics is a term that derives from the Latin *status*, meaning state, and historically statistics referred to the display of facts and figures relating to the demography of states or countries (Bhattacharyya and Johnson 1977). In French, the term *recherche* (research) means to go and look for something. The statistical approach involves defining phenomena in terms of numbers and then using these numbers to either imply or deduce cause and effect. Statistics are a key research tool for quantitative researchers.

Box 2.1 Reviewing

Take a brief look at some quantitative studies. Make a list of (a) the descriptive statistics used and (b) the inferential statistics used. You will find web addresses to articles you can access in many of this book's chapters.

Today statistics are used in a whole variety of studies and investigations. Statistics are used to summarize and describe the data from studies where the data is collected in the form of numbers. Statistics are used to look for patterns and to ascertain the probability of observations having occurred by chance. Statistics are thus a vital tool that underpin all quantitative (number-based) research.

The scientific method

The process of collecting facts in a systematic manner is valued as the basis for the concept of evidence-based practice. This is because, predominately, knowledge for practice is predicated upon the belief that the world and its inhabitants can be viewed objectively, and predictions about things can be proved or disproved. Having a view about how knowledge is created and tested that is shared generally with other people in the world is called a 'world-view' or **paradigm**.

Some beliefs associated with statistics from the quantitative paradigm:

1. Observation and reason are the basis of knowledge.
2. Observations can be numbered, coded, ranked, organized and analysed.
3. Measurements are best made using numbers, as they are unlikely to be tainted by feelings or emotions.
4. Numbers are the best basis for analysing research as they are unlikely to be tainted by feelings or emotions.
5. Individuals are observers of the physical world set on discovering laws that can be used to govern the world and its inhabitants. The rules of the physical world can be represented as universal laws, by which predictions can be made and efforts made to control environments (e.g. the laws of thermodynamics).
6. Individuals of the world respond mechanically to their environment by obeying predetermined universal rules (e.g. touching a hot plate will produce the same reaction in individuals across the world).
7. Reality is not internal to each individual but external to the individual and has an objective nature that can be observed.
8. Events in the world all have causes, which can be discovered through the process of hypothesizing and theory testing.
9. Knowledge exists independently of the individual and is something that can be transmitted and tested for.

Box 2.2 Where do you stand?

Take time to reflect on points 1–9 above; which do you agree with? Are they interconnected? Can you logically agree with some but not all of them?

An alternative view

Whilst this book has a clear focus on statistics and quantitative techniques within research it is worth noting that other forms of data exist. Researchers who use these techniques tend to see the world as socially and individually constructed, with individuals' perceptions and interpretations being the basis of reality. This paradigm is quite different from the quantitative paradigm and has distinctive features.

Researchers who use qualitative data-collection methods view participants as collaborative partners in the research process, who will bring to bear all their biases, variability and individual prejudgements to the data. Qualitative researchers acknowledge this and also acknowledge their own effect on data creation and recognize their 'effect' upon the research co-participants.

Qualitative researchers tend to inform participants in advance of data collection, tell participants what it is they are researching and believe that by being open, honest and reflective about their research the data collected will therefore be more representative of the topic or phenomenon being researched. Qualitative researchers acknowledge and analyse the effect the researcher has had upon the data-gathering process and of working with numerous uncontainable variables.

Qualitative research design is very elastic and flexible enough to pay attention to the multiple sources of participants, of data and potential biases that will inevitably influence the data, once enough evidence has been gathered and analysed to support the case being presented. Qualitative researchers often use techniques such as questionnaires, interviews, focus groups, narratives, historical and contemporary document analysis.

Researchers who gather quantitative data, on the other hand, take steps to eliminate biases and attempt to control as many variables as possible, to try to ensure that data is 'uncontaminated' or unbiased. Some researchers combine qualitative and quantitative data-collection methods; such studies are often referred to as mixed method designs.

The characteristics of research methods that use statistics

Given that quantitative studies tend to have a universal philosophy, they also tend to follow a universal method; this method is commonly known as the scientific method, although it is worth noting that the idea of the scientific method is not confined to quantitative research.

These methods have a number of distinctive qualities, although not all of these will be seen in every study. Studies based on statistics will generally attempt to control the influence of factors (variables) that are not important to the actual study although they could bias the results. All statistical studies rely on evidence derived from observation or experiment as the basis for any new knowledge generated; such information is given the term 'empirical'. An important aspect of empirically based evidence is that it is itself verifiable or provable by observation, experiment and/or replication.

The majority of studies using statistical methods seek to test hypotheses (an idea or theory); by test we mean to disprove (Popper 1959). Thus the studies based on statistics tend to involve the collection of empirical evidence in order to disprove a hypothesis. In general, when using statistics we try to produce results that are generalizable; that is the results from a sample are applicable to the overall population of individuals we are interested in. The link between the sample and the population is the focus of many statistical tests.

Within research the statistical approach is used to:

- describe variables and their relationships;
- help explore the nature of relationships amongst variables;
- help explore the differences between samples and populations;
- help investigate the role of chance in giving rise to measurements;
- help explain relationships between sets of data;
- predict the causes of relationships amongst phenomena;
- control (take account of) variables.

When we examine or establish research using statistics the method used should, more or less, follow the form described below. As it is not the purpose of this book to detail all the research methods, we will not go into the detail of the different aspects of all the methods but focus on indicating where within the research approach adopted statistical analysis lies.

It is possible, for example, to be both analysing data and collecting it at the same time. Indeed, the whole research process should be seen as very dynamic.

Box 2.3   Using studies

Ram Patel works as a nurse in a neurological out-patient department. He is concerned that the level of immediate post-consultation care may be inadequate, particularly in light of the fact that many patients receive disturbing prognoses following their consultations. He decides to embark on a study to assess the impact of the consultation on his patients' immediate health; he intends to use the results to help make a case to increase the allocation of staff to post-consultation care. Ram is aware that he needs to take measures pre- and post-consultation.

1. What quantitative aspects of health could Ram measure?
2. How could Ram use his data as part of an argument to justify more resources?
3. What types of data do you think health care managers prefer to use and why?

Basic parts of the research method

Forming the question(s)

Identify the problem or phenomenon of interest. Decide on the outline of the study, population to be studied and questions that will be investigated. Through searching the literature and drawing on your own thoughts decide on which methods will be used to gather data. At this stage a small pilot study may be conducted that will allow potential problems to be highlighted and obviously if any do come to light there will be a need to revisit the questions being addressed.

The literature review

A vast body of literature that exists concerning many areas of health care; it is essential that any new work is set in the context of any previous or concurrent work. It is also essential that the literature is reviewed so that we can learn from this work before we move on. The literature review will probably start from the moment a research idea is conceived, and it will continue throughout the study.

Conceptual and theoretical frameworks

There are different ways of viewing problems. Many areas of investigation have distinct frameworks and concepts on which the evolution of new knowledge is based. It is important to be aware of these for the particular type of study you are working on. It is likely that a biologist and a sociologist will use different concepts and attribute varying levels of importance to different types of data. Despite having different lenses through which to view the world both these academic disciplines use statistics a great deal.

Hypotheses and variables

In many studies there is a hypothesis; this is a prediction or series of predictions that are under test. Normally the hypothesis originates from a theory. We test hypotheses by measuring relevant variables and investigating how they relate to each other and the populations from which they originate. A variable is a phenomenon (thing) that varies. Not all studies have hypotheses, for example descriptive or exploratory studies.

The research design

The design provides guidelines with which you conduct the research. The design directs the sampling technique and how the data collected is to be analysed. The principal aim of the research design is to minimize all the potential sources of error. It should also strive to ensure that any hypotheses that are under test are actually tested, i.e. the research design should allow the aims of the research to be met. At this stage you must also consider the ethical implications of your work.

Population and sample

The population is composed of all those individuals or objects that you could potentially take measurements from; the sample represents those individuals or objects (given the constraints and resources) that you were able to measure from. Normally we plan to take a sample that is representative of the population being studied. This is subject to the research design being approved by an appropriate ethics committee. You can use statistical techniques to help you to determine the sample size

Data collection

You collect the data, using the method or tool most appropriate.

Data analysis

Here the data are described and summarized, and statistical tests performed. Today, there are many computer-based statistical packages available to help.

Results and conclusions

Having analysed the data you now need to decide what the results are suggesting. You need to decide whether or not any hypothesis under test has been confirmed or rejected. The results need to be related to those from previous studies, and the work needs to be related to an existing body of theory. You should also consider whether you have an ethical duty to communicate the findings of the study.

How do we know if the statistical analysis is any good? Analysing statistics critically

The major concepts involved and the statistical language will becomes more comprehensible as you go on to practise and undertake the exercises at the end of each chapter.

As you become more familiar with statistics you will be in a position to make up your own mind whether you feel a research report that uses statistical analyses is of value. The process to use in making up your mind is the process of getting critical. Getting critical takes a long time, lots of practice and reading of research reports. Do not worry if this seems insurmountable at this stage. Getting critical requires practice and an understanding of statistical concepts.

The process of becoming critical is ongoing and developmental. Once you have tackled an analysis of a research report, your skills will develop and refine. Reading from a wide variety of sources enhances the development of skills for becoming critical. Health care professionals should be encouraged to carry out and critically evaluate research in order to secure the best evidence base for care.

As you go through this book and work through the exercises we hope you will become more critical of how you view statistics. That is to say, we hope you will view all statistics with which you are presented with a healthy degree of suspicion and that your skills and knowledge (enhanced and honed through using this book) will enable you to evaluate if the statistics have been applied appropriately and correctly.

A critical analysis should be considered a balanced evaluation, that is, you need to be aware that a practice theory gap exists even in the field of statistical analysis, which means that sometimes we need to make compromises.

Before starting an evaluation you will need to remind yourself of the steps in the research process and refer to the appropriate chapters in this book. A very important point to remember when carrying out an evaluation is that just because research is published it does not guarantee that the results of an investigation are either valid or reliable. This is ever more so given the large amount of information published on the web.

In Appendix 1 we present a framework that can help you evaluate the statistical components of research and other reports; do bear in mind that there may be other aspects of the research as well as the statistics that you might like to focus on. When evaluating statistical aspects of research reflect on why statistics are used (see above). You can use Appendix 1 to help you practise to become critical; we suggest that you start using Appendix 1 once you feel you have become more familiar and content with the basic concepts of statistical analysis.

Having read this chapter and completed the exercises, you should be familiar with the following ideas and words:

- statistics;
- the 'beliefs' of quantitative research;
- the research method;

- the components of the statistical approach;
- the basis of analysing statistics appropriately.

Select three research papers that report quantitative research.

1. Identify where the steps in the scientific method lie within the paper.
2. Decide whether the papers follow the 'beliefs' outlined in the list of beliefs above.
3. At this stage, how do you feel about the conclusions that the authors reach and the implications for practice? What would you require before implementing a change?

EXERCISES

3

Measuring, sampling and error

Areas of learning covered in this chapter

- What are populations, samples, variables and measures?
- What types of measurement scale and error are there?
- How do scales of measurement influence how I handle my data?

Whilst this book is not about research design it is impossible to learn about statistics without at least knowing something about samples and populations. This chapter will take a look at the concept of the sample and the population.

Population

A population is made up of all the individuals or objects or phenomena that you could potentially measure/count as part of your study. If, for example, you were studying the reasons why nurses in the UK left the profession early your population would be made up of all the nurses in the UK who had left the profession early.

If, on the other hand, you were studying the reasons why nurses in a particular hospital left the profession early your population would be those nurses who left early in that particular hospital.

It is also important to note that the population that we are interested in may not be exactly the same as the one we end up sampling from. This is because some of the individuals within the population of interest may refuse to take part in our study. Thus there may be a distinction between the target population and the actual population.

Sample

In most cases it is unlikely that you would be able to gather information from all the population: you probably would not have the resources. So instead we must take a sample. A sample is made up of a proportion of individuals or objects from the total population available. Many of the statistics described in this book concern establishing how good the sample is at representing the population and whether or not different samples come from the same population. When you read research articles or review numerical data always consider whether the sample is representative of the population being studied. In Chapter 8 we discuss several ways in which poor sampling can mislead people.

There is a great deal of literature that is concerned with how to ensure that a sample is representative; however, as this book is primarily about statistics we will not discuss them here, but we strongly advise that you read around this topic before embarking on any research. A useful chapter to read is Chapter 6 of Blaikie (2003).

Cases

Every sample is made up of the individuals or objects under study. These individuals or objects may be referred to by a variety of names, such as sampling units. For each individual or object we will measure some variable or variables; these variables may be physical (e.g. blood pressure), represent thoughts or feelings (e.g. anxiety) or represent events in the individual's life (e.g. number of visits to a health clinic). The important thing about these variables is that they are measurable. If a variable isn't measurable it can't be dealt with statistically. Each individual or object from which we take a measurement is termed a **case**.

Box 3.1 Measurements and samples

Go to a library or the internet and find five articles. For each decide on:

1. the measurement;
2. the variable being measured;
3. the population;
4. the sample;
5. the sampling unit.

For each case the measurement may referred to as a value. A collection of values is called data.

For every case we should be able to state: the measurement, the variable being measured, the sampling unit, the actual sample and the population being studied.

(Continued)

(Continued)

For example, say we were studying hypertension in populations living near ironworks. Our **measurement** would be 80 mm Hg, the **variable** would be diastolic blood pressure, the **sampling unit** would be individuals that are in the vicinity of the ironworks and the **sample** would be made up of those individuals from whom measurements were taken. The actual **population** is thus defined as all individuals willing and able to be measured living within the vicinity of the ironworks. (Note the exact meaning of vicinity would be determined by the researcher.)

Statistical and real population

In the example above there is a slight difference between the population defined and the one that we originally intended to work on. The defined population includes the term 'willing and able'; obviously you can't take measurements from those not willing to take part in your study. Thus, there can be a difference between the population from whom the measurements were sampled, often called the statistical population, and the real population or biological population, i.e. all those in the vicinity of the ironworks. So beware, not all individuals in a population are available to become sampling units. In some instances, what constitutes the sampling unit and the variables being measured is not at first obvious – look at the examples in Table 3.1.

As you can see from Table 3.1, the range of variables you can use is quite wide; you will also notice that some variables can be expressed as numbers on a scale, whilst others such as gender are discrete. This distinction is very important: before you can identify an appropriate statistical test you must identify the type of variable and on which type of scale it is measured.

TABLE 3.1 A range of different variables and their likely sampling units

Variable	Sample	Sampling Unit
Occurrences of MRSA on a ward	Wards which record occurrences of MRSA that you collected data from	Ward
Length of stay in hospital	Hospitals that record length of stays that you collected data from	Hospital
Pulse rate	Individuals that you record pulse rate from	Individual
Gender	Individuals whom you recorded the sex of	Individual
Hospital position in league table	Hospitals used to formulate league table	Hospital
Number of live births	Units of area from which records of live births have been collected	Unit of area

Measurement scales

Variables can be measured on a number of different scales. Three main types can be recognized: (1) nominal; (2) ordinal; and (3) interval/ratio scales. These will now be discussed further.

Example from the literature 3.1   The population and the sample

Throughout the 1990s, the HOT study group published a series of studies known as the HOT (Hypertension Optimal Treatment) studies, e.g. Kjeldsen et al. (1998). These studies, as the name implies, sought to identify the optimum treatment for hypertension (high blood pressure). Kjeldsen et al. (1998) can be found at: http://hyper.ahajournals.org/content/31/4/1014.full.

The HOT studies were extraordinarily large studies, involving a total of 19,193 participants, from 26 countries, and made up of individuals from different races and genders, and aged between 50 and 80. Individuals with hypertension were included in the study if they were willing and regardless of whether or not they had previously been treated.

The population for this study comprised all those individuals who suffered from hypertension, who presented, who were willing to join the study, lived within the countries participating and were under the care of a practitioner who had subscribed to the study.

The indirect inference within this study is that such a population is representative of the wider global population of individuals with hypertension. The difficulty with this inference of course is that even a study of this size does not cover all contexts (e.g. poverty levels) in which hypertension occurs; in addition, as with all participation-based studies, inference to a wider population makes the assumption that those individuals who agreed to take part in the study had similar characteristics (mental and physical) to those who refused.

The principal variables of interest in this study were diastolic and systolic blood pressure; the sampling is as discussed above.

When reviewing this article do remember it is quite old, and the practice may have been superseded by now.

The nominal scale

The nominal scale is the lowest on the scale hierarchy. Statisticians refer to a hierarchy of scales, because each scale further up the order contains the features of those below. As the name implies, the data occur in named groups; data are classified into the groups. The groups are mutually exclusive: an item of data can't be in more than one group. A good example of a nominal variable is gender.

Ordinal scale

Ordinal scale data is similar to nominal scale except that the names of the group contain an idea of rank or position. A good example here is the grades of staff nurses within a health service; the names of the groups, such as 'staff nurse', 'charge nurse' and 'matron', convey an order or rank. The rank, however, does not suggest how much higher or lower the ranks are. The scale is used to arrange the measures from lowest to highest, but we wouldn't say that a charge nurse is two times higher than a staff nurse. Ordinal scales can be expressed in terms of names, as in the example here, as numbers, such as first and second in a race, and as letters, such as in the UK's old system for grading nurses, i.e. A-I.

Box 3.2

For each of the variables in Table 3.1 state which scale you think that the measurement would be made on.

Ratio/interval scales

In these scales ranks are used but this time the distance between the ranks is known and the distance between the scales is known. The points between the ranks can be subdivided. An example of an interval scale is the centigrade scale for measuring temperature. Ratio scales are similar to interval scales except that they have a true zero point.

If you recorded temperature on the centigrade scale you would know, for instance, that the difference between 37°C and 38° C is 1°C, but the centigrade scale does not have a true zero point so it is not possible to say that 10°C is twice as hot as 5°C.

Box 3.3

For the articles you selected in Box 3.1 now decide which measurement scales they have used. Remember a study may use more than one measurement scale.

An example of a ratio scale is weight; weight does have a true zero (you can't weigh nothing!). Many measures of biological phenomena are measured on either the ratio or interval scales.

You should practise identifying appropriate scales. As you read on in the text you will soon recognize that the choice of statistic and statistical test to use is largely determined by the scale upon which a variable or set of variables were measured.

Example from the literature 3.2   Measurement scales

Looking at the study described in Example from the literature 3.1 above, it is possible to see some of these measurement scales in action. For example, gender (expressed in terms of percentage of males) is measured using a nominal scale (either male or female) as is whether or not participants have diabetes. On the other hand, many of the other variables are measured on ratio scales. No variables were measured using an ordinal scale.

Errors

Although in this book we do not largely concern ourselves with research design, it is important to think about how errors get into our studies. Indeed, a number of statistics that we shall discuss are really about taking error into account. When you conduct a study error can occur in a number of different ways. Statistics can be used to account for or assess some of this error but not all. We will look at three types of error that you need to think about when either conducting your own research or thinking critically about other people's studies. All studies have errors associated with them, the more error that is present the less you can rely on the study.

Measurement error

Measurement error occurs when we try to measure things; this is because most of the tools we need to use to measure things with are not 100 per cent accurate. Even if we are considering something as simple as recording the number of patients who turn up at a doctor's surgery or making a measurement with a ruler, measurement errors will occur.

Consider, for example, making measurements of the length of index fingers using a ruler that is divided using a centimetre scale only. When taking the measurement it would be difficult to record it with a greater accuracy than 0.5 centimetres; a finger that was 5.75 cm long may be recorded as either 5.5 cm long or 6.0 cm long and thus this study has a measurement error. We could then move up and use a ruler with a scale that included millimetres. This would give us a more accurate measure, but for a finger that is 575 mm long, we still need to judge if it is 575 mm, 576 mm or 574 mm long, thus we still have an error, albeit much smaller. Some people will say that the measurement is 575 mm, others 576 mm and yet others 574 mm. This type of error is measurement error. Measurement errors occur in most studies even when the variable is simply a count of something; the counter often makes errors.

Box 3.4   Measurement error

Try measuring the length of the index finger from a sample of ten individuals. First use a ruler marked off in centimetres, then use a ruler marked off in millimetres.

- Which set of measures shows the greatest variation (number of different values)?
- What does this tell you about how useful the different rulers were?

Measurement errors may be **systematic** or **random**. A random error occurs by chance and there is an equal chance that it will be either higher or lower than the 'true' value. Random measurement errors that are sufficiently small are not a significant issue. Sufficiently small measurement errors are those that are considerably smaller than the overall variation in the data. Systematic errors, on the other hand, are those that are consistently either smaller or higher than the 'true' value. Factors likely to lead to systematic errors need to be considered at the design stage.

To deal with measurement errors you need to be aware of them. You should then choose a measurement tool that gives you the greatest level of accuracy, although you will need to consider the resources available to you. For example, high accuracy may involve spending more money or time. If you are using surveyors or interviewers make sure that you train them to use the tools, e.g. the questionnaire.

Consistency

You also need to be aware that some errors will occur because measurement tools are not consistent. For an individual item under measurement an instrument (e.g. a peak flow meter) will not always consistently produce the same measurement, thus instruments need to be calibrated (measured against a known standard) before they are used. You also need to measure how consistent your instruments are between measurements, and between the individuals using the instruments; then you can be aware of this error when discussing your results.

Box 3.5   Are your friends consistent?

Measure out five lengths of string; each should be a different length. Now stand about 5–10 metres away from a friend and ask them to guess the length of each of the bits of string. Show your friend one bit of string at a time. Now repeat until you have data from between five and ten of your friends.

Now look at your results – do some of your friends always overestimate or underestimate the length of the string? What type of error is this?

Do some of your friends seem to overestimate and underestimate in roughly equal proportions? What type of error is this?

Associated with consistency of instruments is consistency of the humans involved in taking measurements. This is known commonly as inter-rater reliability.

As we all know, humans are fallible and as such where we are involved in recording measurements we are likely to make errors and be inconsistent. Take as an example the recording of accidents in factories: some individuals report all accidents however minor, whilst others will only record very serious accidents. Hence if you were conducting a study on reported accidents this inconsistency would introduce error into your study. When counting things, we are inconsistent; what is more, some people are more consistent than others, thus elements of consistency must be considered in any study at the design stage. If you are using several individuals to collect data you must look at each individual to see if they are consistent with respect to themselves and with respect to other researchers. Thus consistency of measurement can be considered both a phenomenon of measurement and design.

Design error

Design error occurs, as the name implies, because the design of the experiment is flawed. There are of course varying degrees to which a study can be flawed and most studies are flawed in some way. If the design error is large, however, then the study will need to be abandoned. This is why it is so important to get the design right. This book is not about research design methods but about statistical analysis. It is important, however, that you are aware of some of the errors you are likely to come across.

The most common error is that the sample is not drawn truly randomly from the population. Thus, the conclusions drawn are not appropriate for the population as a whole. Often, particularly within research related to nursing, studies are based on single sites. This makes it difficult to draw general conclusions that unfortunately authors of such research often do. For example, a study of the performance of nurses in a particular hospital is likely to be biased by that hospital's working environment; it is unlikely that the results would be generalizable either nationally or globally.

The second most common error is to fail to take into account **extraneous variables**. Extraneous variables are those variables that, although not of interest, may alter the value of the variable being measured (often called the **dependent variable**). You may be able to control (hold constant) some of these extraneous variables. Time of day, light levels, temperature, health status of participants, sex of participants and age of participants are all examples of variables that could influence the results of various studies; with careful design these variables cam be eliminated as sources of error.

Besides controlling for the extraneous variables another important technique used is to measure the extraneous variables and take into account their influence on the variable of interest statistically. For this technique advanced statistical tests need to be used, and these are beyond the scope of this book. One problem the researcher cannot account for is those extraneous variables that they may not be aware of before the start of the study. This is a surprisingly common problem and although such problems can often be overcome, the best solution is a thorough reading of the research literature and careful design, and even then the problem can still arise.

Box 3.6

For each of the articles you used for the exercise in Box 3.1 suggest what:

1. measurement errors have been made;
2. design errors have been made.

For each article reflect on whether they have discussed these errors and how they impact on the conclusions.

Sampling error

Sampling error is the error that many statistical techniques try to take account of; sampling error is the difference between the sample and the population. If we take a sample it is unlikely that the measures taken from the individual of this sample will exactly match that of the population. When we look to see how representative a sample is of the population or whether or not two samples come from the same population we need to take into account sampling error. Sampling error will increase the more variation there is amongst the sample you are measuring and decrease as the sample size increases.

The relationship between sample size, sample variation and sample error is important because one question you are bound to ask is 'How large should my sample be?' and the answer is, it depends on the variation within the sample.

If you were working with the variable height using a population of professional basketball players the variation in height of this population would be very small, and thus the sample size that you require would be small. If, however, you are working on the variable height across the global population the variation would be large and a larger sample would be required.

Having read this chapter and completed the exercises, you should be familiar with the following ideas:

populations;   measurement error;
samples and sampling;   design error;
scales of measurement;   sampling error.
consistency;

EXERCISES

1. For each of the studies below, indicate (a) the variable being measured, (b) the sampling unit, (c) the sample, (d) the statistical population:

    (i) a study on the impact of exercise on the bone density of women aged between 35 and 45;
    (ii) a study on the different rates of outbreak of meningitis in villages in the south-west of England.

2. For the study on sexual health presented in Chapter 5 describe (a) the population and (b) the sample.
3. For the study on sexual health presented in Chapter 5 identify for four of the variables (a) the scale it is measured on and (b) the measurement error that could be associated with it.
4. Summarize what you understand by the term 'sampling error'.

4

Questionnaires

Areas of learning covered in this chapter

- What are questionnaires used for?
- How are questionnaires designed to avoid bias?
- What types of questions can I use?
- How do I ensure that a questionnaire is reliable and valid?

Introduction to questionnaires

We have included a chapter on questionnaires because we recognize that many health-related research studies use questionnaires as a data-collection tool. However, the subject of questionnaires and research design is huge and cannot be addressed in detail in one chapter of a text this size. We aim to provide an overview and highlight some of the important considerations about the formulation, distribution and use of questionnaires as a method of data collection and statistical analysis. A useful textbook about questionnaires is Oppenheim (1992). A really good background account of the development of questionnaires and the history of their various designs can be found in a textbook by Burns (2000). A useful guide to developing questionnaires can be found in Gillham (2008).

The term **questionnaire** usually means a form containing a set of pre-determined questions used for gathering information (data) from and about people as part of a **survey**. The term 'survey' is used to describe a research approach that attempts to cover as wide a range of the population as possible in order to obtain information about a subject or topic area.

Questionnaires can be used in various types of research, such as descriptive, comparative and attitudinal. There are many different types of questionnaire. The type of questionnaire used will depend on the research question being asked. Questionnaires can be used to produce both qualitative and quantitative data, and can be used:

1. as a means to describe a population;
2. to investigate cause and effect (see Chapter 9);
3. to monitor change over time in, for example, a **longitudinal** study.

Often questionnaires attempt to describe a population's behaviour, its attitude or commonly held view, with regard to a certain topic, or understanding of an issue or level of understanding. Surveys often use questionnaires in order to obtain such information. Sometimes an interviewer may also be used.

Questionnaires can be used to provide information from people on a particular topic and can use two main types of question options. First, open questions, meaning the person completing the questionnaire is free to put in their own thoughts, views and responses (or not as they see fit). Second, closed questions, meaning the answers are constrained to a particular range of answers predetermined by the researcher. The questionnaire described below uses closed questions; this type of questionnaire lends itself to statistical analysis as the answers can be pre-coded and then loaded onto a computer program, for counting and preliminary analysis. Open questions need to be analysed using techniques for analysing **qualitative data** and as such are beyond the scope of this book.

Box 4.1   Questionnaire design

Three of the main questions to ask when thinking about designing a questionnaire are:

- What is it that I wish to find out?
- Is it to do with knowledge or attitudes or levels of understanding, or is it about behaviour or activities or decision making?
- Why is a questionnaire the best option?
- Can a questionnaire really measure the phenomenon I am interested in?
- How will I administer the questionnaire?
- How will I distribute the questionnaire – by hand, by post, by email or as a web-based form?

In questionnaire designs the perspective of the researcher is important to ascertain, as it provides clues as to the kind of relationship the researcher has with the individuals they are collecting questionnaire data from and the questions they have asked. Questionnaires which ask for a numerical response are sometimes considered (as we have done largely) as quantitative instruments; in fact, in all but the most simple questionnaires there is always a qualitative element that takes place when the questionnaire is designed.

A very helpful and informative textbook that discusses the background and detail of the main types of questionnaires used in quantitative research is Burns (2000); see also Oppenheim's (1992) invaluable and seminal text.

When used as a quantitative data-collection tool, questionnaires help to put numerical indicators on these phenomena. As a quantitative research tool questionnaires are a good method of collecting data, although such data can tend to be superficial, as there is no room for probing or extracting the meaning of the responses. Questionnaires are a cost-efficient way of collecting large quantities of data in a short space of time, and if the questionnaire is properly structured large quantities of data can be collected and subjected to statistical analysis. Once a questionnaire is constructed, it is usually referred to as an instrument or tool. The methods by which questionnaires can be administered include not only face-to-face interview but also telephone, mail, e-mail and web based interviews, making this method of data collection attractive to researchers doing large-scale, international research.

Sample questionnaire

In Box 4.2 we describe a questionnaire that could be used to ascertain some aspects of the sex-related behaviour of a group of people. (Please note that the full questionnaire is given in Chapter 5.) Let us say, for example, you wanted to know more about the epidemiology of AIDS and HIV in the UK. It might be useful to know more about the general sexual health of the population in the UK. Safe sex is much discussed in the media and has recently been the cause of major concern in Public Health England, when reviewing the evidence of rising rates of sexually transmitted diseases (STDs). One reason is that many more older people (over fifty) are discovering new-found sexual freedom following easier divorce proceedings and a more liberal attitude to recreational sexual activity. One way of keeping safe during recreational sex is to use barrier methods of contraception. Large amounts of money are spent by governments on health promotion programmes to educate the general population about safe sex.

A survey using a questionnaire could be used to give an indication of the nature of sexual activity within this group and others. Once devised, the questionnaire is distributed to a sample of sexually active adults in the UK to find out what types of sexual protection (condom, femidom or dental dam) are used. This kind of survey would try to establish when people used protection, when they were least likely and most likely to use protection, and how much money was spent on sexual protection per week. The information might be useful in a health promotion context:

- if running a safe-sex campaign in a family planning clinic or in a genito-urinary clinic;
- when identifying specific health promotion needs used in identifying trends in patient/client behaviour;
- when considering social policy issues relating to such health issues as national trends in the development of STDs and HIV/AIDS.

Initially, the population that is to be sampled must be targeted, for example consenting adults over the age of eighteen years. Note that this would not give you any information about those under eighteen, as they are not part of the target population.

Box 4.2 The questionnaire

This survey is attempting to find out about the use of barrier methods of contraception/protection. Your answers will be treated in confidence and will help us plan health care services.

Please indicate your responses by placing a cross in the box next to the answer you think *best represents your answer.*

(1) strongly agree, (2) agree, (3) not sure, (4) disagree, (5) strongly disagree.

1. I use the following types of barrier protection:

	Always → Never				
	1	2	3	4	5
None	□	□	□	□	□
Condom	□	□	□	□	□
Femidom	□	□	□	□	□
Dental dam	□	□	□	□	□
Cap (Dutch cap)	□	□	□	□	□

2. When are you most likely to use sexual protection?

	Agree → Disagree				
	1	2	3	4	5
I never use barrier methods of sexual protection	□	□	□	□	□
I sometimes use protection when I remember	□	□	□	□	□
I use a condom every time I have anal penetrative sex	□	□	□	□	□
To avoid pregnancy	□	□	□	□	□
Allergic to latex	□	□	□	□	□
To avoid getting a sexually transmitted disease	□	□	□	□	□

3. Please indicate your circumstances: which of the following categories applies to you?

Single
Married
Living with spouse
Living with partner
I have many sexual partners
I have one sexual partner

Thank you for completing this questionnaire. Please return it in the enclosed pre-paid envelope. Your responses will be treated in confidence.

Questionnaires: the reality

A common misconception about questionnaires is that they are often considered an easy tool to use in research. In reality, the use of questionnaires requires a great deal of time and effort in terms of careful planning, ordering and sequencing of the questions and the responses in order to obtain relevant data. As with most research, we need to address questions of design early in the research design. When using questionnaires not only do we have issues of the sample to consider (see Chapter 3) but also specific issues that concern the questionnaire, for example:

- When should the questionnaire be administered and how: by mail, in person, by telephone interview or face to face, e-mail or internet?
- Where should the questionnaire be administered and by whom?
- How will the questions be arranged in terms of sequencing, degree of ease or difficulty?
- Are the questions to be addressed in the questionnaire intrusive, do they pry into sensitive or private areas of people's lives, such as death and dying or sexual persuasion or activities, and are they likely to cause offence or distress to respondents?

The importance of the points raised above is that they all have the potential to bias the answers that you receive. If for example you are asking questions about sexual behaviour, whether you use telephone or face-to-face questioning is likely to alter the results, as is the gender of the respondent in relation to the interviewer. Any bias will introduce error, which will make interpreting the results harder.

In addition to the considerations above you will need to think about how the information will be handled and stored, remembering that many countries have laws to protect respondent or subject confidentiality and the use to which data can be put. This is also important for all types of research where personal data are collected. Many countries have specific legislation that covers how data can be stored and how they can be used. You must make sure that your systems of data handling conform to the law of whichever country you are working in.

When we want to use a questionnaire to produce quantitative data it is important that all our variables and the responses are given in a form that can be analysed using statistics. This means that the answers should come in the form of numbers. If you intend to use a computer to help with the analysis it is also important for the variables to be given codes that the computer finds easy to handle. When preparing data for analysis each case should be given a row on a table and each variable a column (see Table 5.1). Most data from questionnaires tend to be either ordinal or nominal scale data.

Asking questions

When designing a questionnaire there are also issues concerning the formulation of the questions. You need to consider how the questions will impact upon the answers.

Box 4.3 Leading questions

Try asking your friends or colleagues how they rate the quality of their lunch. Can you lead them to suggest in general their lunch is (1) poor or (2) good? Which types of question are the best at leading?

Look at the sample questionnaire. Which of the questions do you think are leading? How would you rephrase them?

Leading questions

A leading question is a question that leads the respondent to a particular answer. By using leading questions experimenters have been able to demonstrate effects on guessing measurements, past personal experience and recently witnessed events. In everyday language we often use leading questions, and as such, when designing questionnaires, leading questions are often easy to include by mistake. Things to watch out for in particular are an implied direction when asking a respondent to put a value on something. If we were to ask people to indicate their degree of agreement with the statement 'Condoms are a good form of contraception' more people would tend to agree with the statement. If, however, we asked the same people to indicate their agreement with the statement 'Condoms are a poor form of contraception' we would also find more people tending to agree with the statement. In both cases we have led the respondents to the answer. Emotive words should also be avoided. Studies have shown, for example, that when people were asked to estimate the speed at which two cars collided, the actual speed suggested depends on the word used (smashed, crashed, etc.) to describe the collision.

Ordering

Care needs to be taken when ordering questions; in general, the basic principle is that the ordering should be logical and that the questionnaire should appear structured and clear. For example, if you were asking people about their experience as a diabetic it would not be logical to ask questions about how they delivered insulin before asking if the respondents were insulin-dependent. Structure can be achieved through grouping similar questions together, either by subject or by type of answer.

Box 4.4 Writing questions

- Develop five questions using a Likert scale to measure the quality of health care service used by your peers.
- Ask at least three of your peers to respond to the questions you have devised and ask each to indicate to you how clear they think the questions are.
- Do you need to revise the questions?
- Did the questions you asked appear to measure what you intended?

Sensitive questions should be placed towards the end of the questionnaire, as they can cause people to refuse to answer. An early refusal tends to lead the respondent to abandon the questionnaire.

Example from the literature 4.1   Designing an effective questionnaire

Do not be under any illusion: designing an effective questionnaire is not easy. Reading Castle's (2004) paper explains how a questionnaire to evaluate family satisfaction with nursing care will give you a good impression of the work involved. Do not worry about how the questionnaire's psychometric properties are explored (unless you are interested); it is relatively complex and beyond the scope of this text book. Box 4.2 gives the details of the questions asked; do you think any of them are leading? The article can be found online at: http://intqhc.oxfordjournals.org/content/16/6/483.full.pdf+html

---

Questions about the respondents' personal details should also come at the end. Asking for this information at the start tends to make respondents concerned about your commitment to their confidentiality.

Scales

When asking respondents a question we quite often give them a range of options so that they can indicate where their answer lies according to a scale. In the example questionnaire above (Box 4.2) we used a scale for respondents to express their frequency of use of differing types of contraceptive and also a scale for respondents to indicate their level of agreement with certain statements. There is a range of scales of this type; we will now discuss three of them.

The scale most commonly used with questionnaires is a Likert scale, named after Rensis Likert, who invented it. Likert scales are based on multiple questions that are based on the extent to which a person agrees or disagrees with the question. The most common scale is 1 to 5. Often the scale will be (1) strongly disagree, (2) disagree, (3) not sure, (4) agree and (5) strongly agree.

One common problem with using a scale which is based on an odd (five) number of options is that it always provides the option of choosing the middle point. Often it is easier for respondents to take this 'easy' option than to struggle to make a decision. Using a scale with an even number of options (four or six, for example) forces respondents to choose between tending to agree or tending to disagree. There are two problems here. Some individuals may be genuinely neutral, and using an even number of options forces on them a choice they may not agree with; and psychologically individuals may assume that the scale has a 0. Thus if you present a scale of 1–4, people will select 2 as a neutral value, as on a normal number line 2 is half-way between 0 and 4. In general it is probably better to opt for an odd number of options and accept that those people who select the neutral option probably do not have a strong opinion.

Another type of scale is the Thurstone scale. A Thurstone scale uses just two points: agree and disagree. When using Thurstone scales, it is usual to ask several related questions that can

TABLE 4.1 A patient's responses when asked to consider day surgery (questions asked pre-operatively)

Exciting	1	2	3	4	5	6	Boring
Frightening	1	2	3	4	5	6	Calming
Useful	1	2	3	4	5	6	Useless
Fast	1	2	3	4	5	6	Slow

be used to produce an overall score for an individual respondent. The overall score can then be compared with that for the sample as a whole, or used so that differing populations are compared. A common example of the use of Thurstone scales is in psychometric tests. Psychometric tests measure aptitude and attitude. You might expect to complete such a test as part of a job interview.

An alternative approach is to use semantic differential scales, which are good for investigating phenomena such as attitude and values. A semantic differential scale is based on opposite points of view, or potential emotions about a subject or concept. The respondent is asked to indicate where on the scale he or she sits. We may, for example, be investigating people's work environment. We ask questions concerning how they felt about aspects of the environment, and the response scale may range from helpful, nurturing and happy to unsupportive, blocking, toxic and dysfunctional.

In Table 4.1 the concept is 'day surgery'; patients are asked to indicate where on the scale they lie. You would probably want to ask more questions to get a good overview of an individual's impressions of day surgery. Note that there is no consistent negative end of the scale. This helps to persuade the respondents to think about their answers.

Validity and reliability of questionnaires in statistical analysis

Questionnaires should be seen as measurement tools, just as we view a thermometer or a ruler. As with these tools, we need to ask about the validity of the measures – do they really measure what we think they do? – and reliability – will the same result be returned over time and if administering the questionnaire were to repeated?

With questionnaires, rather than dealing with the validity and reliability of instruments, the issues centre on the interaction of the tool with individuals, whose responses can change depending on their circumstances. Unlike the measurement of physical responses, the types of circumstances and level of impact are not easy to measure, and much effort needs to be devoted to ensuring that a questionnaire is reliable and valid. As this book concerns quantitative analysis, below we explore the concepts of reliability and validity as they relate to the quantitative analysis of data from questionnaires.

Reliability

Reliability involves two main concepts: consistency over time (or stability), for example if you record results from one group of individuals do you get the same results if you measure the same group a few days or weeks later, and will these results demonstrate internal consistency? This means, will this questionnaire produce similar responses under repeated conditions?

To test for stability (consistency over time) it is possible to perform a reliability re-test to show the extent to which the same scores are obtained when the instrument (questionnaire) is used with the same subjects twice. This test produces a **reliability coefficient** that indicates how small the differences are between the scores. The coefficient ranges between 0.00 and 1.00, the higher the score the better.

The internal consistency relates directly to the way in which the questions in the questionnaire design measure an attribute consistently and nothing else. This means that all the items on the scale are accurate in their focus on the phenomenon of interest. Similar respondents will tend to give the same pattern of answers if the questionnaire is internally consistent. If we introduced a question that had little to do with the other questions, the internal consistency would decrease. For example, if in the survey on sexual health we introduced a question such as 'To what extent do you agree with the statement "Ice cream is nice"?' we would not expect the answers to be at all related to respondents' previous answers and therefore internal consistency would be lost.

There are various methods of determining internal consistency. The most common is the **Cronbach alpha reliability coefficient** test. Again the coefficient ranges between 0.00 and 1.00, the higher the score the better. In general, a score above 0.80 indicates a high level of internal consistency. The score's value is, however, related to the number of questions asked. As you ask more questions the score will tend to increase.

Validity

Validity refers to the extent to which a questionnaire measures what it is supposed to measure by obtaining data relevant to the topic which is being measured; for example, if the topic area for measurement is degrees of sexual libido, how can degrees of libido be measured whilst ensuring that measuring deviance or sexual perversion does not become the focus of the research? There are several different forms and measures of validity. We discuss some of these below.

Content validity

This is a weak form of validity and concerns the **representativeness** of the questions; in other words do the questions adequately sample the content being investigated? One way to ensure that questions asked of respondents are valid, pertinent and measurable is to conduct a thorough literature review of the topic before constructing the questionnaire.

Face validity

This is obtained through asking a member of the lay public to assess questions for accuracy and completeness. If you want to assess whether the content reflects the subject matter, you can use a panel of experts or a group of peers. This is often termed a *focus group*, as the panel or group shares the same focus of interest in the topic being investigated.

Criterion-related validity

This is a strong form of validity, as criterion-related validity measures the ability to compare equally to another already validated measuring instrument or questionnaire. This instrument has shown itself to be accurate in obtaining or measuring data.

Predictive validity

This refers to the ability of the questionnaire to predict some criterion observed at a future date with the data collected on the criterion variable at a different time but on the same subjects, for example school results and end-of-year university examinations.

Construct validity

This is the most difficult type of validity to achieve. The question is: what construct is the instrument actually measuring? The more abstract the construct the harder this is, because of the absence of objective criteria to measure the construct, for example grief, role conflict, empathy.

Known-groups technique

This means you can use two groups who have a shared experience in whom you would expect to see a difference, for example measuring fear of childbirth in pregnancy. You could, for example, choose a group of primaparas and a group of multiparas. Your guess or research hunch is that the first-time-pregnant group is more likely to express fear of the labour process than those who have had several births. This may be reflected in the scores.

How can questionnaires be analysed?

Having obtained your data, you will want to analyse it. Most phenomena measured by questionnaires use either the **nominal** (categories) or **ordinal** scales (see Chapter 3), and these will affect the type of descriptive and analytical statistics that you can use. Chapter 6 discusses how data measured on the ordinal scale can be described and Chapter 7 how they can be displayed. Chapters 14 and 15 describe statistical tests that are particularly useful for the type of data gathered by questionnaires.

Having read this chapter and completed the exercises, you should be familiar with the following ideas and concepts:

- when to use a questionnaire;
- types of question not to ask;
- basic aspects of questionnaire design;

- the concept of reliability;
- the concept of validity;
- response scales.

1. For the research on the walk-in clinic presented in Chapter 5, review the questions and decide which, if any, are leading. How would you improve on this questionnaire?
2. Identify three research studies from the literature that use questionnaires. For each research (a) decide what the research question was and why a questionnaire was appropriate, (b) review how the validity and reliability of the questionnaire were considered.
3. Using a topic that interests you, draw up a short (six questions) questionnaire using questions that are not leading. Ask a colleague or friend to assess the quality of your questions. Do they lead? Are they clear and unambiguous?

5

The studies

In this chapter, we provide the background and data from two hypothetical studies, one from a clinical trial and the other from a questionnaire. In some of the exercises at the end of each chapter, we ask you to analyse data from these studies. If you work your way through all the exercises you will have completed a basic analysis of these data sets and be able to draw some conclusions and be in a better position to critique this and other studies. These studies have been devised to be relevant to modern health care as well as to stimulate your interest and enjoyment of data analysis. Please note the main purpose of this questionnaire is to provide data for you to analyse; therefore we have not presented data from all sections of the presented studies.

The questionnaire study

This questionnaire concerns the sexual health of individuals who presented for advice at a walk-in clinic in central London. It was partly introduced in Chapter 4. Here we show the extended version.

The aim of this study is to provide basic information as to the sexual behaviour of individuals of differing sex, age and ethnic group who used the walk-in clinic. The study was initiated because the clinical leader considered that a large **proportion** of the clients were presenting with symptoms that related to sexual heath and she is considering putting in a bid for funds to support the employment of a specialist in this area. The study is largely descriptive and exploratory in nature.

The intended population of the study is all those individuals who could potentially use the walk-in centre. The sample is made up of those that actually do enter the clinic and complete the questionnaire.

The questionnaire

This survey is attempting to find out about the use of the walk-in clinic in relation to sexual health. Your answers will be treated in confidence and will help us plan health care services. Please indicate your responses by placing a cross in the box next to the option you think best represents your answer.

1. What made you attend the walk-in centre today?

Agree ————————————→ Disagree

	1	2	3	4	5
Location	☐	☐	☐	☐	☐
Availability	☐	☐	☐	☐	☐
Access to medical staff	☐	☐	☐	☐	☐
Access to nursing staff	☐	☐	☐	☐	☐
Emergency treatment required	☐	☐	☐	☐	☐

2. What symptoms are you experiencing? Please tick the ones that best describe your symptoms.

Headache
Chills/shakes
Temperature
Lack of appetite
Feeling generally unwell all over
Cough
Pain/soreness in chest
Faintness
Collapse
Pain or difficulty passing urine
Discharge from penis
Discharge from vagina

3. Which of the following descriptions best represents your sex life? (Please tick.)

(a) Very active (I have sex more than five times per week)
(b) Active (I have sex between once and five times per week)
(c) Not very active (I have sex less than once per week)
(d) Non-existent

4. Please indicate how many sexual partners you have shared sex with in the past month.

5. My most frequent choice of barrier protection is: (Please tick one.)

None
Condom
Femidom
Dental dam
Cap (Dutch cap)

6. When are you most likely to use sexual protection?

Agree ——————————→ Disagree

	1	2	3	4	5
I never use barrier methods of sexual protection	☐	☐	☐	☐	☐
I sometimes use protection when I remember	☐	☐	☐	☐	☐
I use protection (put a condom on) if I do not know my sexual partner very well	☐	☐	☐	☐	☐
I use protection (put a condom on) when I think I am going to climax	☐	☐	☐	☐	☐
I use a condom every time I have oral sex	☐	☐	☐	☐	☐
I use a condom every time I have vaginal penetrative sex	☐	☐	☐	☐	☐
I use a condom every time I have anal penetrative sex	☐	☐	☐	☐	☐
To avoid pregnancy	☐	☐	☐	☐	☐
To avoid getting a sexually transmitted disease	☐	☐	☐	☐	☐

7. What puts you off using sexual protection?

Agree ——————————→ Disagree

	1	2	3	4	5
Not very comfortable	☐	☐	☐	☐	☐
Loss of sensation/cannot feel anything	☐	☐	☐	☐	☐
Too fiddly to have to open packets	☐	☐	☐	☐	☐
Cost	☐	☐	☐	☐	☐
By the time the packet is open the moment has gone	☐	☐	☐	☐	☐
Need to use a lubricant as well	☐	☐	☐	☐	☐
Have to plan sex in advance	☐	☐	☐	☐	☐
Allergic to latex	☐	☐	☐	☐	☐

8. How much money do you spend on average on sexual protection per week? Please indicate which category applies to you using a tick.

£0

£0–£5

£5–£10

£10–£15

I get them free from a family planning clinic

9. What is your age?

10. I consider my sexual orientation to be:

heterosexual male
heterosexual female
gay (homosexual) male
gay (lesbian) female
bisexual male
bisexual female
virgin

11. I consider my ethnic background to be:

a) African
b) Asian
c) European

NB: This questionnaire has been simplified for the purpose of this book.

TABLE 5.1   The data from the questionnaire

Individual	Sex Q13	Ethnic group Q12	Sexual activity Q3	Partners Q4	Barrier choice Q5	Reason Not Q7	Presentation Q2	Age Q9
1	F	E	3	1	1	1	1	22
2	F	E	2	2	2	5	7	28
3	F	E	1	8	2	7	4	21
4	F	AS	2	1	2	1	9	26
5	F	AS	4	O	O	5	12	27
6	F	AS	2	1	O	7	6	30
7	F	AS	4	O	2	5	5	29
8	F	AS	2	2	O	5	12	23
9	F	E	4	O	1	3	10	21
10	F	E	2	1	O	2	9	32
11	F	E	1	1	1	2	3	18
12	F	E	1	1	3	7	10	24
13	F	A	1	3	5	6	12	23
14	F	A	2	4	1	1	7	23
15	F	A	1	1	5	3	12	20
16	F	A	3	O	2	5	1	36
17	F	E	1	4	O	5	2	20
18	F	E	3	1	O	1	5	23
19	F	E	4	O	2	3	3	24
20	F	E	4	2	3	3	3	20

(Continued)

TABLE 5.1　*(Continued)*

Individual	Sex Q13	Ethnic group Q12	Sexual activity Q3	Partners Q4	Barrier choice Q5	Reason Not Q7	Presentation Q2	Age Q9
21	F	E	3	O	2	1	12	34
22	F	E	3	1	1	7	12	25
23	M	E	1	12	2	4	2	19
24	M	E	2	1	1	6	1	53
25	M	E	3	2	2	3	1	26
26	M	A	2	1	2	4	5	29
27	M	A	3	2	1	4	7	58
28	M	A	3	2	1	2	7	37
29	M	A	1	12	O	5	8	22
30	M	A	2	3	1	4	11	23
31	M	A	4	1	O	4	3	36
32	M	A	2	1	1	5	8	25
33	M	AS	2	1	2	6	12	44
34	M	AS	4	1	2	6	11	41
35	M	E	2	1	2	6	2	22
36	M	E	4	1	1	4	8	27
37	M	E	1	18	2	8	11	35
38	M	E	2	2	1	1	11	35
39	M	E	2	2	1	8	7	22
40	M	E	1	1	1	2	8	39

When entering data into charts and computers it is often easier to use a line for each participant and enter values across the rows for the variables measured. Often codes will be used to simplify the data entry. In Table 5.1 we have used the following codes:

For gender we have used 'M' for male and 'F' for female.

For sexual activity we have used a codes 1–4 where 1 = very active and 4 = non- existent.

For 'Barrier Choice' we have used codes 1–5 for the most used protection the participant selected where 1 = the first response possible (i.e. none) and 5 the last (i.e. Cap).

For question 7 we have used a similar system to that used for barrier choice where 1 = the first option and 8 = the last option.

For the presentation type we have also used the same system as for questions 5 and 7, with 1 = 'Headache' and 12 = 'Discharge from vagina'.

The clinical trial

This experimental trial looks at the ability of the novel drug Symphadiol, designed to help increase weight loss, in individuals who are trying to lose weight using a calorie-controlled diet. This clinical trial is being organized by Spinto, a drugs company who are active in this field. Spinto have recruited individuals to take part in their study using a network of dieters' groups. Individuals were invited to take part by Spinto's clinical trials specialist nurse who will conduct the study, with the support of local GPs and Spinto's dietician.

The aim of the experiment is to test the hypothesis that a daily does of Symphadiol enhances weight loss in clinically obese individuals, compared with just using a calorie-controlled diet. It was decided to select men between the ages of 30 and 40 for the study. It was also decided to look at the impact of exercise in conjunction with Symphadiol.

The intended population of this study are all healthy (other than their obesity) obese male individuals who are sufficiently motivated to lose weight to join a diet network. The individuals must not be taking any medication, except that required for minor ailments.

In total 60 males were recruited between the ages of 30 and 40. Each participant was given a health check prior to the start of the study, their heights were recorded and they received educational material and diet plans giving details of a calorie-restricted diet (2000 kcal), which they declared they would follow. All the men attended weekly diet networks where they received support and encouragement from their fellow dieters and the clinical trial specialist nurse. Those individuals following an exercise regime also attended a gym and completed the equivalent of 30 minutes cycling (16 km) three times per week.

The 60 participants were distributed randomly to four experimental groups:

group 1: calorie-controlled diet and **placebo**;

group 2: calorie-controlled diet and Symphadiol;

group 3: exercise regime, calorie-controlled diet and placebo;

group 4: exercise regime, calorie-controlled diet and 35mg Symphadiol.

Table 5.2 shows the results for sixty of the participants, fifteen from each group.

TABLE 5.2 The data from the clinical trial

Individual	Age	Height (cm)	Group	Weight loss (kg)
1	32	159	1	23
2	35	174	1	16
3	35	188	1	28
4	33	174	1	12
5	30	195	1	8

(Continued)

TABLE 5.2 *(Continued)*

Individual	Age	Height (cm)	Group	Weight loss (kg)
6	38	195	1	17
7	39	176	1	−1
8	36	193	1	16
9	31	159	1	20
10	38	170	1	1
11	33	177	1	6
12	38	167	1	7
13	34	184	1	−3
14	37	193	1	10
15	39	181	1	14
16	31	186	2	23
17	32	182	2	18
18	36	158	2	8
19	38	170	2	12
20	31	184	2	15
21	36	176	2	0
22	35	158	2	1
23	30	169	2	9
24	34	175	2	16
25	37	188	2	15
26	37	188	2	10
27	34	195	2	6
28	37	182	2	4
29	34	171	2	0
30	38	198	2	18
31	32	181	3	20
32	34	169	3	13
33	34	181	3	22
34	34	190	3	24
35	37	193	3	23
36	30	177	3	11
37	35	158	3	10
38	35	181	3	18
39	37	181	3	18
40	37	183	3	25
41	25	176	3	7
42	35	172	3	11
43	38	192	3	18
44	35	194	3	20
45	30	179	3	14
46	35	171	4	25
47	38	179	4	27

Individual	Age	Height (cm)	Group	Weight loss (kg)
48	36	178	4	28
49	31	188	4	17
50	33	180	4	21
51	35	184	4	13
52	37	173	4	5
53	39	176	4	5
54	38	170	4	6
55	32	190	4	26
56	32	152	4	6
57	37	182	4	10
58	35	175	4	10
59	34	180	4	8
60	32	162	4	22

Please remember that these studies are hypothetical and are designed to help you practise. As with all skills if you don't practise they won't develop. Use these data how you wish, discuss your results with colleagues and have fun.

6

Descriptive statistics

Areas of learning covered in this chapter

- How are data described and summarized?
- What are measures of central tendency and dispersion?
- How are measures of central tendency and dispersion calculated?
- Which measure of central tendency to use and when.
- How to calculate an odds ratio.

We use descriptive statistics when we want to describe what our data looks like or what its most common features might be. Descriptive statistics are used to summarize our data. After all, if you were to present all the data that was gathered in a study, your audience would probably soon lose interest and more importantly not be able to follow your results or believe your conclusions.

Descriptive statistics are used to give the reader a summary of the data you have collected. Producing descriptive statistics will also help us to understand whether we have captured the sort of data we want. For example, using the variable 'age' descriptive statistics could demonstrate whether we had captured the range of ages we wanted, or had accidentally include too many young people or perhaps a few people in the sample were much older than the rest of the cases in the sample. Descriptive statistics allow us to get a feel for the data, to appreciate its common features and any unusual features. This is nothing new; we do this to understand behaviours and actions all the time. For example, a common question on lifestyle surveys is to ask how much time you give to exercise in a day; obviously you are not expected to write that on Tuesday you spent forty minutes, Thursday thirty-seven minutes, etc. It will expect you (or even ask you) to give an average. Say, for example, on average you exercise forty-five minutes a day. But some days when you are tired you may exercise for just twenty minutes, while on a particular energetic day you may do eighty minutes. Then you would have exercised anywhere between twenty and eighty minutes. In this example the researcher is asking you to summarize your day-to-day exercise level and provide a descriptive statistic, the 'average'. Descriptive statistics allow us to summarize detailed data in a manner that can be interpreted quickly and easily.

Descriptive statistics are used in many aspects of health care; they are in fact the most common type of statistic you are likely to encounter. Descriptive statistics are used to manage, to monitor and evaluate health services and the people that work within those services. This is why understanding descriptive statistics is so important for those who work in a health setting.

Box 6.1 Descriptive statistics

Think about the statistics that you have heard or seen in the last week.
Why do you think they were quoted?

Descriptive statistics are usually separated into two types:

1. measures of central tendency (typical value), for instance the mean, mode and median;
2. measures of variability about the typical value (measures of dispersion), such as the range, inter-quartile range, **standard deviation** and variance.

Measures of central tendency

Mean

The arithmetic **mean** is usually called the average. To calculate the average time we spend in a gym in a month we would take the times spent during each visit, add them together and divide by the number of visits.

Table 6.1, for example, displays the time that an individual (Mr Armstrong) spent in the gym during the month of July.

TABLE 6.1 Time spent by an individual at the gym during July

Visit	Time Spent (minutes)
1	62
2	34
3	50
4	40
5	58
6	48
7	38
8	60
9	58
10	45
11	53
12	32

To calculate the mean:

Minutes spent in each visit

$$Mean = \frac{32+34+38+40+45+48+50+53+58+58+60+62}{12} = \frac{578}{12} = 48.16$$

Total number of visits

So, the average (mean) length of time spent in the gym is 48.08 minutes. You can see that this score of 48.16 minutes falls exactly in the centre of our data with six visit times less than this and six greater. This is, however, not always the case with the mean.

Unfortunately for those just starting out in the world of statistics, being a branch of mathematics often statistical tests are represented as a formula. Understanding them is like learning another language. It is the use of these symbols which usually makes people convinced they cannot understand statistics. So to introduce a few:

Box 6.2 Calculators

Most statistics involve only the use of calculations that can be carried out on a basic calculator. Most calculators also have a facility that will allow you to perform the basic statistical calculations faster, and once data sets become large use a computer package. Look on your calculator for some of the symbols described below. If your calculator has a statistical function, it normally can be found below the function buttons.

x an individual case like one visit to the gym

n the number of cases (x) so twelve visits to the gym means that n = 12

Σ means the sum of, e.g. all the xs added up, in the case above Sx = 578

$\bar{x}$ is the symbol for the mean

Another way of describing how to calculate the mean other than using words is:

$$\bar{x} = \frac{\Sigma x}{n}$$

(Note this is the formula used when calculating the mean for a sample from a population.)

If you have problems following a statistical formula write out each symbol in words, thus for the mean we have:

$$mean = \frac{the \quad sum \quad of \quad the \quad cases}{the \; number \; of \; cases}$$

There is, however, one disadvantage with the mean: it can be misleading when some of the data are unusually small or large. If, for example, Mr Armstrong on one extra day stayed in the gym for just five minutes, adding this value to our data will affect the average score making the average 44.85 minutes.

Box 6.3

In the example from the gym, the sample is one month's visits; the population would be all of Mr Armstrong's visits. When dealing with whole populations statisticians use different symbols to distinguish between samples and populations. In addition, when calculating statistics, the equations slightly change. This book will focus on statistics that concern samples from populations, but do be aware that there are subtle differences.

Some symbols used when talking about populations

N the population size

μ the population mean

σ the standard deviation (see below) of the population

5, 32, 34, 38, 40, 45, 48, 50, 53, 58, 58, 60, 62

↑

44.85

Box 6.4   Calculators (again)

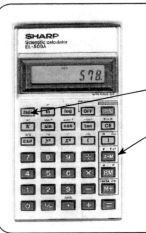

On this calculator, statistical functions can be accessed through pressing the second F key and then the ON/C key. Down the left-hand side you can see the statistical functions available. Look for some of the symbols we have discussed.

When you go shopping for a calculator, we suggest that you look for a basic scientific calculator that has at least one memory storage and of course statistical functions. We don't of course have space in this book to explain how to use your calculator, but most come with manuals and, with help from friends, all will become clear.

You can see how this unusual score of 5 has made the mean about 10% lower; therefore it is not a true reflection of the central point. These extreme values are called outliers or outriders.

Median

The median helps to solve the problem of outliers because rather than use all the values to calculate the statistic of central tendency it uses only the value that sits in the middle of the data. It is the physical centre. So far we have put our data in ascending order. This is essential to do when calculating the median.

If we take our two examples of exercise time and include the low value, we can see that they have very little impact on the median even when they only occur at one end.

$$32, 34, 38, 40, 45, 48, 50, 53, 58, 58, 60, 62,$$

↑

Median = 49

$$5, 32, 34, 38, 40, 45, 48, 50, 53, 58, 58, 60, 62,$$

↑

Median = 48

The extreme value only moves the median by 1. Where the middle falls between two values, it is necessary to add the two middle numbers and divide by 2, e.g. $\dfrac{48 + 50}{2} = 49$

Box 6.5

Collect a sample of the pulse rate from fifteen individuals:

1. Calculate the mean.
2. Calculate the median.

So why don't we hear or see the median being quoted more often? The simple answer is it is not widely understood by the general public but also because the median is not arithmetically based it cannot be easily manipulated or used in further calculations

Mode

The **mode** is the most frequently occurring value, so from our data set we can see it is 58.

$$32, 34, 38, 40, 45, 48, 50, \mathbf{53, 58}, 58, 60, 62,$$

The mode shows the most common value. One of the advantages of the mode is that it can be used on both continuous and nominal data whereas the mean and median can only be used on continuous data.

At times, therefore, it is the only option as a measure of central tendency. For example, one question a lifestyle survey asked was where students would primarily go for family planning advice.

TABLE 6.2   Sources of family planning advice used by a sample of students

GP	Practice nurse	Family planning clinic	Friends	Chemist	Nowhere
5	4	6	8	2	2

So the most commonly occurring category was friends, with eight scores. For the data in Table 6.2, the mean and median would have no meaning (pardon the pun).

Choosing a measure of central tendency

It is most common to use the mean as it is the most sensitive. The mean considers all the values of each case in the distribution, as described above, and it is arithmetically based, so it can be used in further calculations. However, it can only be used on data of interval or ratio level of measurement and is easily distorted by outliers.

The median which does not take account of the values of the cases is unaffected by outliers and is suitable for ordinal/ranked data. Where the mean is distorted by the presence of outliers, the median should be used.

Box 6.6   Choosing measures

Ask a sample of your friends how often (each week) they eat chocolate. For this sample, find:

1. the mean;
2. the mode;
3. the median.

Which do you think best represents the typical value and why?

The mode can be used on data of all levels of measurement but is most useful for categorical data. On a normal distribution, the mode, median and mean should all be the same. It is also possible to have more than one mode.

In many circumstances, there is no right or wrong measure of central tendency and people tend to opt for the arithmetic mean because they are familiar with it. Remember the main point of descriptive statistics is to communicate information. You should choose the measure that conveys the information in the best possible way and does not mislead the audience.

TABLE 6.3   Choosing a measure of central tendency to use

Measure	When to use	When not to use
Mean	Interval or ratio data	Categorical data
	For most data sets, where the cases are more or less symmetrically distributed about the mean.	Ordinal data
		When there are outliers or data is heavily skewed
	Where the measure is going to be used in further calculations	
Median	Interval, ratio or ordinal data	When measure will be used in further calculations
	Data heavily skewed, mean distorted by outliers	Ordinal data
Mode	Categorical	Ordinal data

Measures of dispersion

So far we have looked at central values. Now we are going to explore statistics, which tell us how different our scores within a sample are. Dispersion is the term given to those measures that tell us about the level of variability with the data. If there were no variation in populations there would be little need for statistics.

We asked two groups of students, one full time and one part time, how old they were when they had their first sexual experience with another person.

Group A $14, 15, 18, 22, 23 = \bar{x}_A\ 18.6$

Group B $17, 18, 19, 19, 20 = \bar{x}_B\ 18.6$ This sub-script tells us that the mean is that of group A

Whilst the means are the same it is obvious that there is a difference in the variability of the values of the cases with the groups.

In terms of using the statistics to develop health care practices, knowing the variability of values is as important as knowing the mean. After all, if shoe manufacturers only made shoes for people with average-sized feet they would soon go out of business. We want to know about the variability that we will encounter in patients' health and in their behaviours.

One measure of dispersion is the range; to calculate this you subtract the lowest score from the highest, so:

The range of group A is $23 - 14 = 9$
The range of group B is $20 - 17 = 3$

This tells us that for group A scores are spread over nine units, but for group B, they cover only three. This means that group A has a greater range of values in their cases.

The range is a quick and easy way of estimating the level of variation within your sample, but beware of outliers.

In the following example, we asked a group of teenagers for how many years they thought it was safe to take the oral contraceptive pill.

$$Q_2$$
$$2, 2, 4, 5, 8, 10, 10, 10, 12, 15, 15, 30$$
$$Q_1 \qquad Q = \text{quartile} \qquad Q_3$$

The range is 28 but it is affected by the case with the value of 30.
The inter-quartile range is the first quartile minus the last $= 12 - 4 = 8$

In the case of outliers in ordinal/ratio level data, the median was used in preference to the mean; in this case, a variation of the range is adopted. This is called the inter-quartile range (IQR). A **quartile**, as the name suggests, is derived by quartering the data set. The data are placed in ascending order and divided into four quarters. The numbers at the boundaries form the quartiles.

The IQR overcomes the problem by ignoring the extreme values. However, we cannot elect to ignore just the outliers as this would distort our data (and is known colloquially as fiddling your figures); we have to deal with each end of the data line in the same way, and thus we can produce values for the, lower middle and upper IQRs.

Box 6.7

Calculate the IQRs for the data you gathered for the exercise in Box 6.6.

Whilst the range and IQR say something about spread, they ignore any concept of the level of deviation from the central tendency. The standard deviation (SD), however, uses each score to calculate spread and how far each score is, in standard terms, away from the mean.

The standard deviations and variance

The two most common measures of dispersion that indicate the amount of deviation from the mean are the standard deviation and the variance. Most quoted in describing data is the standard deviation, whilst the variance is used in many statistical tests.

The standard deviation is a measure of the variation in the data that evaluates how much each case deviates from the mean. If the mean is say 6 and an individual case is 8 then the deviations is 2. Whilst this is easy enough and takes care of the deviation part of the statistic it's really the standard bit that is important. To obtain a standard deviation we take all the deviations and look at them in relation to the size of the mean; this is important because a deviation of 2 is of much less importance if the mean is 110 than if it is 8.

The formula for the standard deviation is given below. It looks complex but it really involves quite straightforward maths. We will take you through the formula step by step using the data in Table 6.4.

$$s = \sqrt{\frac{\Sigma(x - \bar{x})^2}{n-1}}$$

s is the symbol for the standard deviation and s^2 is the symbol for the variance. The variance is simply the standard deviation squared.

TABLE 6.4   Age at first sexual experience (with another person)

Case	1	2	3	4	5	6	7	8	9	10
Age of first sexual experience	14	15	17	18	18	19	19	20	22	23

The calculation steps are outlined below:

1. Calculate the mean.
2. Subtract the mean from each value $x - \bar{x}$.

$$
\begin{array}{llll}
14 - 18.5 = & d1 & -4.5 \\
15 - 18.5 = & d2 & -3.5 \\
17 - 18.5 = & d3 & -1.5 \\
18 - 18.5 = & d4 & -0.5 \\
18 - 18.5 = & d5 & -0.5 \\
19 - 18.5 = & d6 & 0.5 \\
19 - 18.5 = & d7 & 0.5 \\
20 - 18.5 = & d8 & 1.5 \\
22 - 18.5 = & d9 & 3.5 \\
23 - 18.5 = & d10 & 4.5 \\
\end{array}
$$

d stands for difference

$\Sigma d = 0$ (taking into account the signs)

21   (ignoring the signs)

3. Square each answer obtained in step 2.
4. Add up all the answers to step 3 squares; this value is called the sum of squares.
5. Minus 1 from the size of your sample $n - 1$.
6. Divide the value found in step 4 by the value calculated in step 5.

$$
\frac{\Sigma(x - \bar{x})^2}{n - 1} = \frac{70.5}{9} = 7.83 \text{ this is called the \textbf{variance}.}
$$

7. Find the square root of the value obtained in step 6 to determine the value of 1 standard deviation. $\sqrt{7.83} = 2.80$

Thus, the standard deviation of our sample was 2.80.

Box 6.8 Standard deviation

We asked a group of thirty people to keep a record of how many times they thought about sex in a day. The results were 7, 7, 8, 10, 10, 12, 14, 15, 16, 17, 18, 20, 20, 21, 21, 21, 22, 23, 24, 26, 28, 28, 30, 32, 34, 35, 36, 38, 40, 42.
Is the mean a good measure of central tendency and how spread out are the results from it?

If you want to do a statistical test be cautious of data sets where the square of the standard deviation (the variance) is much larger than the mean (two times) or where the variance is small in relation to the mean, or where the variance equals the mean. These are indications that the data set might have a more complex form and need to be handled in a particular way.

It is important that when you quote a mean you should always give a measure of the dispersion. A measure of the mean without a measure of dispersion is difficult to interpret; the sample

TABLE 6.5 Common measures of central tendency and dispersion

Type of data	Measure of central tendency	Measure of dispersion
For most data sets, where the cases are more or less symmetrically distributed about the mean	Mean – there should be no need to quote any other measure because all measures of central tendency for this type of data will be similar	Standard deviation and also consider giving range
Interval, ratio or ordinal data	Median, although you might also quote the mean	Range and quartiles
Data heavily skewed, mean distorted by outliers		
Nominal	Mode	No measure

size should also be included. Remember these important facts when you next hear the average house price or salary quoted in the press or on TV.

Which measure of dispersion should you quote? In general, when you use a mean give a standard deviation; if you quote the median give the inter-quartile ranges. Don't be modest with your use of measures of dispersion; remember descriptive statistics are about describing your results to your audience.

Percentages, proportions ratios and odds ratios

Without doubt, one of the most common descriptive statistics you will hear is the percentage, probably rapidly followed by proportions. In the health care services you will often find that percentages are used to summarize management information such as the percentage of beds used in a hospital at a given time and for information such as the proportion of clients with particular conditions or issues. Proportions and percentages and ratios are also used to express phenomena such as the chance of an individual surviving or becoming pregnant or to describe the sociological make-up of particular communities.

A percentage is really a particular method to express a ratio; for example if there were forty women in a class and twenty men we could say that the proportion of females in this population is two-thirds. Alternatively we could calculate the number of females as a percentage of the total which would be approximately 66.6 per cent. We could also say in terms of a ratio that two in every three people in this population is a woman. Thus, it is possible to see that all these types of measures are connected and can be used to express data where we want to compare the amount of one thing to another.

Sometimes when percentages or proportions are used they can lead to misdirection; this is because they are summaries of raw data. With questionnaires, for example, you may find quoted that 80 per cent of people strongly agree with a particular statement; a closer look, however, may reveal that just five people completed the questionnaire. Thus, it is becoming normal to report such data as the raw value followed by the percentage in parenthesis, in this case '4 (80 per cent)'. Further examples of how statistics can potentially mislead are given in Chapter 8.

Odds ratio

Odds are the chance (i.e. probability) of something happening expressed as a proportion. The odds of something happening can be calculated as the number of times that something happened divided by the number of times it didn't if given the opportunity. The chance of you tripping on a particular paving slab could be estimated from the number of times individuals have tripped on that paving slab whilst walking over it divided by the number of non-trips.

In more health-related terms you may want to ask what is the chance of a smoker getting lung cancer. For the sake of discussion let us say that it is 1 in 5. In other words of five smokers, one is likely to develop lung cancer. Now this data may be useful, but it does not tell us the potential risk of smoking because at present there is nothing to compare it with. To make such data really useful we need to compare the odds of the smoker getting lung cancer with the odds of the non-smoker. To do this we need to calculate the odds ratio, that is the ratio of one set of odds with another.

An odds ratio is normally calculated by dividing the odds in the 'exposed' group by the odds in the non-exposed group. Again for the sake of this discussion let us say that the odds in the non-smoking group are 1 in 20. In other words, of non-smokers 1 in 20 is likely to go on to suffer from lung cancer. The next step is to convert the odds from the exposed group into a decimal. So 1 in 5 becomes 0.2 (1/5) and to do the same with the non-exposed group, thus 1 in 20 becomes 0.05(1/20). To compare the ratios we divide the value for the exposed group with that for the non-exposed giving 0.2/0.05 = 4. Thus in our hypothetical example the smokers are four times more likely to develop lung cancer than non-smokers. Odds ratios are becoming a more commonly used descriptive statistic and are discussed further in Chapter 18.

Having read this chapter and completed the exercises, you should be familiar with the following ideas and concepts:

- describing data using statistics;
- measures of central tendency;
- the appropriate use of the mean, median and mode;
- how to calculate the mean, median and mode;

- the terms 'dispersion' and 'variation';
- the appropriate use of the range, quartiles and the standard deviation;
- how to calculate quartiles, standard deviation and the variance.

EXERCISES

1. For the study on the walk-in clinic presented in Chapter 5 calculate the mean, median and mode for the data on number of partners. (a) What is the most appropriate measure of central tendency? (b) What do these results suggest?
2. For the study on Symphadiol presented in Chapter 5 calculate the mean, median and mode for the data on the weight loss of each of the individuals in the study. (a) What is the most appropriate measure of central tendency? (b) What do these results suggest?
3. For the data in Exercises 1 and 2 above, calculate the quartiles and standard deviation. Discuss which type of measure of dispersion you feel is most appropriate. What do these measures tell you about the data?
4. Find five examples where a descriptive statistic has been quoted. For each example decide whether the measure is appropriate. Discuss the measures of dispersion used with the measure of central tendency.

7

Displaying data

Areas of learning covered in this chapter

- What are the various ways of displaying data?
- How do you choose an appropriate way of displaying your data?

This chapter will explore some of the ways that data can be displayed. It provides a rationale for the choice of display and how display type is linked to the type of data.

The two most common forms of data display are graphs and tables. Both have the same aim, to summarize and present the data in a manner that is easy to understand and take in. Displaying your data is an essential part of analysing the data; it allows you to establish how the data are distributed, to see unusual cases and generally get a 'feel' for the data.

Tables present information in a text-based form; as such much of the detail in the data can be retained. Unfortunately taking in lots of different numbers and seeing emerging patterns is rather difficult and this is where graphs come in. When we present data in graphical form some of the detail tends to be lost but it becomes much easier to see the emerging patterns. In the example below we show some data from a study by Acklin and Bernat (1987) in graphical and in table form. Acklin and Bernat's (1987) study examined the relationship between chronic low back pain and depression. In the graph and the table, we have taken two of the indices of depression that they used and plotted them against patient type.

Box 7.1 Rules

1. Provide legends for tables and graphs.
2. Categories and values must be clearly identified.
3. Note units of measurements for interval/ratio data.
4. Indicate total number of units.
5. Identify source.

TABLE 7.1   Acklin and Bernat (1987) data for two indices of depression measured in patients with a range of conditions

Indices	Patient Type			
	LBP	Depressives	Personality Disorder	Non-Patients
Egocentricity index	0.31	0.32	0.42	0.39
Sum morbid content	0.82	3.47	0.99	0.70

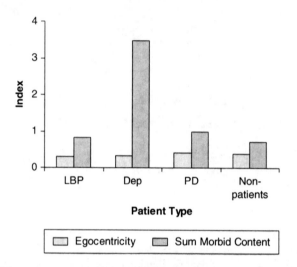

FIGURE 7.1   Indices of depression recorded by a range of different patient types (Acklin and Bernat 1987)

Which display form makes it easier to see the trend? Which allows you to see most detail? As a general rule the more data put into a table the more it will become harder to read, and less likely to be read. Tables should be used when the data set is very simple or when you need to show your data in great detail. The data we used for these graphs are already summaries of the data collected. This means that the figures are averages.

Table types

There are several different table types that can be used. Your choice of table will depend on the type and number of variables that you have. In the example in Table 7.1 there are two types of variable: along the top of the table we have the nominal category 'patient type', whilst down the side of the table we have two interval scale variables, i.e. the indices of depression.

Other tables may have just one variable, which runs either along the top or down the side of the table. The measurement could be the frequency or occurrence of that particular variable. In such a case the table becomes a 'frequency table' and it is normal to have the most commonly occurring frequency at the top (see Table 7.2).

TABLE 7.2 Frequency of different ethnic groups of a sample of 178 individuals interviewed in north-east London

Ethnic group	Frequency in sample
White European (EU)	75
African	35
Indian	32
Afro-Caribbean	26
Other	10

Sometimes tables may include summary statistics (as does Table 7.1). In Table 7.3 the bottom row is a summary of the data within the table.

TABLE 7.3 Summary examination results for a group of 122 first-year student nurses

Examination Paper	Percentage (Average)
1	53
2	46
3	58
4	43
AVERAGE	**50**

Tables that report on frequency values of two nominal variables simultaneously and that include totals are often used to help look for associations between variables. These tables are known as **contingency tables** and are discussed in Chapter 16.

Graph types

The guiding principle behind using graphs is that less is more. If too much information is included in the graph the data will not be understood by your audience. All graphs are plotted against two axes, the horizontal axis and vertical axis. The horizontal axis is known as the *x*-axis and the vertical axis as the *y*-axis.

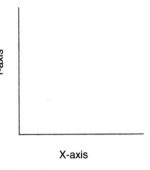

FIGURE 7.2 Horizontal (x) and vertical (y) axes

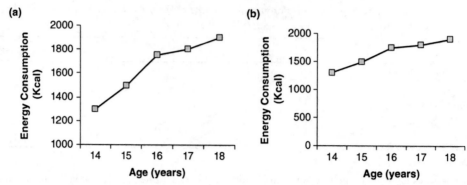

FIGURE 7.3   Energy consumption (kcal) in relation to age for a teenage girl between the ages of 14 and 18: (a) drawn with x-axis starting at 1000 and (b) with x-axis starting at 0

An additional point to consider is that if your graph is drawn incorrectly you may mislead your audience (see also Chapter 8).

Figures 7.3a and 7.3b show the same data. They indicate the average daily kcal. consumption of an individual teenage girl between the ages of fourteen and eighteen. The first graph displays a relatively rapid increase in calorie consumption over a five-year period. In the second example the increase looks much slighter. This optical illusion is caused because in the left-hand graph the y-axis starts at 1000 whilst in the right-hand graph it starts at 0.

Sometimes data may be presented in a manner that seeks to use graphical techniques to obscure trends rather than reveal them. Understanding graphs will help you spot this type of presentation.

There are a variety of graph types. The main types you will see are: frequency charts, histograms, bar charts, pie charts, scatter graphs and line graphs. The type of chart that you should use depends on the type and complexity of the data. We will now discuss each of these in turn.

Box 7.2   Axis

- Do not need to start from 0.
- Should increase in units appropriate to the measure.

Frequency charts

We quite often divide data into categories and/or counts of how often a particular value occurred. These counts of occurrence are known as frequencies. The simplest form of data are nominal data where we categorize things, and then count the number of things in each category. Some examples of such categorize are the number of males and females, different types of diseases and number of individuals belonging to each ethnic group. To display such counts or frequencies a form of **bar chart** can be used.

Figure 7.4 shows an example relating the number of visits to an eye clinic and social class.

If these data are measured initially on an interval or ratio scale, the most appropriate form of display is a **histogram**. Plotting data using a frequency histogram allows us to get an idea of how the data are distributed and also to get a 'feel' for the data.

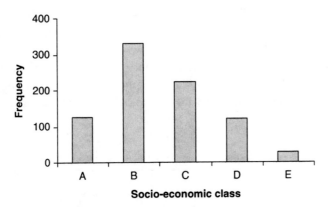

FIGURE 7.4 Comparison of frequency of visit to an eye clinic and socio-economic class

In a frequency histogram, the x-axis covers the range of values of the cases. Each distance covered by a 'bar' on the x-axis represents a range of potential recordable values for the measure. You need to decide the size of the range categories that you will use. If you have too few categories then the detail and patterns will be lost; if you have too many categories, the patterns will be lost

TABLE 7.4 Peak flow (l/s) measurements from 20 males and 20 females

Females	Males
563	654
605	736
631	663
618	717
623	706
657	732
585	661
600	716
574	722
604	718
612	687
622	716
670	714
604	666
612	684
577	729
596	735
684	650
698	683
594	719
Mean 616	Mean 700

in the detail. Once you have decided on the range of each of your categories, you then count the frequency of the number of cases in each range. Then plot a horizontal bar above the range on the *x*-axis at the height on the graph indicated by the *y*-axis.

The *y*-axis displays the number of times (frequency) that a particular case value is recorded. Table 7.4 shows the peak flow rates for twenty males and twenty females. For the data for the males, the range of categories we have used and their associated frequencies are shown in Table 7.5.

TABLE 7.5   Ranges and frequency of peak flow measurements taken from twenty male patients

Range	Frequency
640–660	2
661–680	3
681–700	3
701–720	7
721–740	5

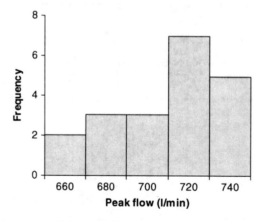

FIGURE 7.5   Frequency histogram of the peak flow measurements of 20 male patients

Pie charts

Pie charts are an alternative form of frequency chart. Pie charts are best used with nominal or ordinal scale data. A pie chart displays the count of things in each nominal group category as a proportion or frequency of the total number of counts. The total data set is represented as a circle; the circle is divided into segments the size of which reflects the frequency of each nominal group. For example, Figure 7.4 shows the results of a survey of the choice of contraception by women (between the age of 15 and 50) carried out by the UK Department of Health in 1999.

Box 7.3 The first?

During the Crimean War, Florence Nightingale recorded the impact of her various interventions on the morbidity of injured soldiers using pie charts. Florence Nightingale's work probably represents one of the first uses of pie charts and of a systematic evidence-based approach to the provision of nursing care.

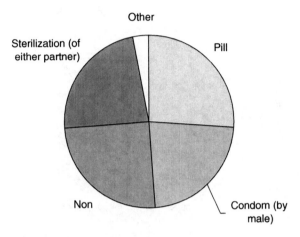

FIGURE 7.6   Pie chart showing choice of contraception amongst women aged fifteen to fifty

Pie charts are ideal for simple data. If you want to divide the data further, say for example you were interested in the choice of contraception by different age groups within the population, then you might want to present a pie chart for each sub-group. The difficulty here is that as you start to use more pie charts it becomes more and more difficult for the eye to make comparisons. As a rough guide, three pie charts should be the maximum – any more and you will make it difficult for your reader. If you want to make comparisons between different categories consider using a bar chart as this makes it easier for the reader (see Figure 7.1).

Bar charts for summary statistical information

Bar charts can also be used to display summary statistical information such as means and standard deviations (Chapter 6). In Figure 7.1 the means of two indices of depression are plotted on a bar chart. We could also plot on the graph an indication of the variation in the data; this is often done in the form of error bars. Error bars are small vertical lines with horizontal bars at the top and bottom that mark the range of the mean ±1 standard deviation or standard error (see Chapter 9). For the data on peak flow, we can show the mean for each gender and give a graphical representation of the standard deviation in the form of error bars (Figure 7.7). This lets your audience see quickly how much variation there is in your samples.

Box 7.4 Remember

1. Bar charts can also be incomprehensible if too many categories are used in stacked bar charts.
2. For nominal and ordinal data there is always a space in between the bar to indicate the scale of measurement is not continuous.

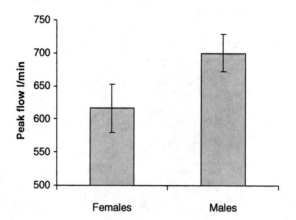

FIGURE 7.7   Mean peak flow for a group of twenty males and twenty females (horizontal bars represent 1 SD)

Scatter graph (scatter plot)

A scatter graph is used where we are interested in whether or not there is an association between two variables, i.e. is the value of one of the variables linked to the value of another, for example weight and height are quite often closely linked. Scatter graphs can be used with interval, ratio or ordinal data that has been collected in pairs (e.g. you have measured both the height and the weight of each of your participants).

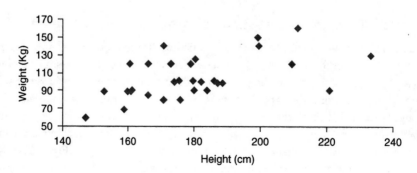

FIGURE 7.8   The relationship between height and weight in thirty white European males

The x-axis carries the scale for one of the variables, whilst the y-axis carries the other. Points are plotted on the graph for each sample unit. A spot is plotted at the point where the values of x and y for a particular sampling unit meet. If you have sufficient data, the graph will show a scatter of points over the surface of the graph, which with a bit of luck may show a trend (Figure 7.8). You may want to fit a trend line to this type of data (see Chapter 17).

Line graphs

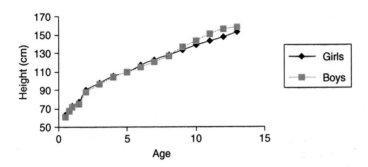

FIGURE 7.9 A scatter plot of height versus weight for a group of European children

A line graph is similar to a scatter graph except that the points are plotted in sequence as the values increase along the x-axis and a line is drawn between each point and the next. Line graphs are ideal for showing sequences, for example plots of patient observations over time, or growth of infants over time. In general, line graphs should be used only when there is a very good reason to assume that the line drawn between the points does really represent what in all probability will happen. As such they should not really be used for grouped data, such as monthly means or counts. Line graphs are quite a good way of allowing comparisons in trends across different groups of data. In the example (Figure 7.9), the height of boys and girls is compared over time.

Presenting data is something of an art. There are some basic rules that help, which we outline in Table 7.6. In the past, it was normal to use pen and paper to produce graphs; now it is much more common to use a computer. We have drawn all the graphs used in this book (with the exception of Figure 7.10) using Microsoft Excel. It is worth noting that the basic unchanged (default) output from many packages used to draw graphs is initially quite poor. You will need to work with the package to produce the output that you want.

Box and whisker plots

When we use graphs and figures we are trying to give the reader a good impression of the data, rapidly and in a simple form. Box and whisker plots are a form of graph that attempt to show both central tendency and a range of measures of central tendency.

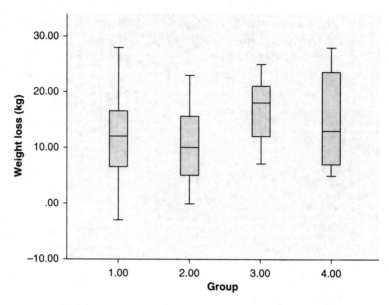

FIGURE 7.10   Box and whisker plots of one of the groups from the Symphadiol experiment (Chapter 5)

They are very useful as a method to give a visual impression of a variety of the **parameters** of your data sets. In the example above we have taken the data from the Symphadiol experiment described in Chapter 5. Each separate box and whisker plot represents the data of weight loss of one of the groups (Figure 7.10).

In box and whisker plots the dark line in the middle signifies the median (as read against the *y*-axis), the horizontal boundaries of each box are the first and third quartiles, and the tips of the whiskers are the range. With the exception of nominal data box and whisker plots can be used with all types of measurement scale, and are a very good way to get a quick visualization of your data.

Examples from the literature 7.1   Graphs

The literature is replete with examples of different ways to display data. The following web addresses lead to health research papers that use a variety of different graphs. Collison et al. (2007) use a scatter plot to illustrate the relationship between mean income inequality ratio and under-five mortality rate in a range of developing nations. When you read this paper, note how they have identified each point on the scatter graph. http://intl-jpubhealth.oxfordjournals.org/content/29/2/114.full

Graphs used by researchers in publications do not always follow a standard. An article from the *Bandolier* on analgesia uses bars to illustrate the Numbers Needed to Treat (NNT – see Chapter 17) vs analgesia type. These bars, however, not only illustrate the

(Continued)

> *(Continued)*
>
> mean NNT, but also the 95 per cent confidence limits. You can find this work at www.medicine.ox.ac.uk/bandolier/booth/painpag/Acutrev/Analgesics/Leagtab.html.
>
> Balcázar et al. (2005) use classic bar charts to describe results from a heart health outreach programme. www.ncbi.nlm.nih.gov/pmc/articles/PMC1364518/ . The work of Caplan et al. (2006) examined an approach to reducing admissions of elderly patients to hospital, using line graphs to illustrate fluctuations in admissions over time. http://ageing.oxfordjournals.org/content/35/6/581.full.

Exploring and describing data

It is important to recognize that plotting data is not just an approach to help others interpret your data; it is also an approach that helps you to understand and interpret your data. So, before you move to analyse your data, plot it in an appropriate form; study the measures of central tendency and dispersion before you go on to do anything else.

TABLE 7.6   Guidelines for drawing perfect graphs

Rules

1. Keep your graph simple, few variables, don't select the complex option.
2. Label axes and variables clearly.
3. Each graph should have a legend – this is a short description of the graph and a reference to the key points and the sample size.
4. Don't forget a key if there is more than one variable or group.
5. Make sure you plot the points accurately – don't use large markers.
6. Choose an appropriate scale – many computer packages will not do this for you, so you will need to practise.
7. Make sure the units on the scale change in a way that suits the data.

Graph Types

Graph type	When to use
Histogram	Used for showing a frequency distribution of data measured on the interval or ration scales.
Bar chart	Use for displaying frequencies of nominal or ordinal data; also use for comparing measures of central tendency between groups for data measured on ordinal, interval or ratio scales.
Pie chart	Used largely for showing the frequency distribution of nominal data. Try to avoid using pie charts to compare between different groups of data.
Scatter graph	Use with interval, ratio or ordinal data when you want to see if two variables are linked. Two or more variables must be measured from each sampling unit.
Line graph	Used for data measured on interval, ratio or ordinal scales, particularly when you want to display a trend or change over time. Particularly useful for displaying trends in several groups of data at once. Do avoid joining points if there is no reason to do so.

Having read this chapter and completed the exercises, you should be familiar with the following ideas and concepts:

- the importance of displaying data;
- how to choose an appropriate display;
- types of table;
- using tables;

- using graphs;
- selecting the appropriate graph;
- bar charts, histograms, pie charts, scatter graphs and line graphs.

EXERCISES

1. From the questionnaire data (Chapter 5) select the most appropriate method to display the numbers of patients presenting (frequency) with each types of symptom.
2. From the study into Symphadiol select and display the data of the mean weight loss from each of the study groups such that a comparison can be made. Include in your display a measure of the standard deviation.
3. Take your resting pulse, and then perform some light physical exercise (be careful if you are not particularly fit). After the exercise, at intervals record your pulse, repeat this five times (record the time interval). Plot a graph showing the change in pulse rate with time.
4. Review three articles that use graphs to display their data. For each decide (a) if the display is appropriate, (b) if the authors followed our rules, (c) how the display could be improved.

8

Lies, damned lies and statistics

Areas of learning covered in this chapter

- What are the ways statistics can be used to mislead?
- How to avoid being misled by poor statistics.

The title of this chapter may seem slightly strange – after all statistics are designed to inform and help to elucidate the 'truth'. Statistics, however, do have a bad press. One of the oft-quoted sayings about statistics is that 'there are lies, damned lies and statistics' (sometimes attributed to Benjamin Disraeli, but the origin is not clear). The implication of this quote is clear: if you want to really deceive, use statistics. In a similar vein and probably more pertinent is the saying: 'A politician uses statistics like a drunkard uses a lamppost; more for support than illumination' (often attributed to Winston Churchill, but more likely to be Andrew Lang). Here again we see the suggestion that statistics are used to persuade, influence and support a position rather than to shed light on the truth. Indeed, we are all used to hearing politicians exchange statistics in order to gain support for their arguments.

The quotations above indicate a general suspicion of statistics within the general population, and that they can be used to deceive, particularly in cases where the intended recipient of the statistics is poorly informed about statistical information and can be easily bamboozled by statistical presentations.

Early history of statistics

The early history of the use of statistics reveals they are often used as tools of government. Early definitions of the word 'statistics' refer to their purpose as being able to describe 'states', i.e. countries or units of government, the data collected being largely either demographic (about the number, gender, age and location of a population) or economic (as in gross domestic product). *The Domesday Book*, an inventory of settlements in England, published in 1086, is an early example of a collection of statistics being used to describe the current level of 'assets' within a country. *The Domesday Book*, in part, was used to help determine levels of taxation, which was often inappropriate to the relative wealth of individuals or communities or commensurate with their ability to pay taxes. With these types of misuse by governments it is hardly surprising that statistics have a 'bad press'.

Statistics in health care

Health care practice is replete with statistics as statistics are used internationally, compiled by organizations such as the World Health Organization (WHO) at national levels to determine the distribution of health care resources, for example to General Practitioners in the UK to spend on health agencies and primary and secondary care and to determine health care need. At a local level they are used in the management of the organizations that deliver health care, for example as measure of efficiency and efficacy such as **metrics** in hospitals. Statistics are used to determine which treatments and therapies are the most appropriate and/or most cost effective to use by agencies and organizations such as the National Institute for Clinical Excellence (NICE), who also research the risk associated with various available treatment protocols and approaches and even to determine the risk associated with not intervening. The association between statistics and health care is not new. In 1662 John Graunt published a summary of the *Bills of Mortality*. Bills of mortality were weekly reports on deaths and causes of deaths in London. The 'bills' had been formulated since the end of the sixteeenth century. Graunt used his analysis of causes of death in London to identify health issues and suggest solutions to some of London's most pressing social problems that caused early deaths; in other words, to help formulate heath care policy to tackle the reduced life expectancy of Londoners.

The extensive use of statistics within health care together with the mistrust of statistics within the general population has the potential to generate difficulties for health care professionals, for example if patients/clients are asked to believe the information that they are given regarding their health care intervention. Patients and clients need to be advised appropriately and to make informed decisions about their treatment and health. It is important that health care professionals are able to interpret, understand the significance of and be able to criticize the statistics they are using and make informed decisions if the statistics are credible (or not). Health care professionals need a critical eye to determine how and which health care management statistics are collected as critical analysis of statistical data can help avoid expensive management mistakes.

The aim of this chapter is help you to develop a critical approach to the statistics that you encounter in your daily practice but in particular it will examine the ways in which statistics or more accurately the presentation of statistics can be used to mislead the unsuspecting reader. It is important to remember that it is not that statistical data 'lies' but the way in which statistical data is (mis)used, combined with a lack of critical enquiry from those using the statistics, that leads to misunderstandings and misrepresentations. The power to be misled by statistics is reduced by having an ability to understand and be critical of statistical data and analysis.

This chapter will be confined largely to the ways in which statistics and the outcomes of investigations can be presented and described in such ways that an audience might be misled.

Research studies using statistics can generate misleading results for a number of reasons; for example, poor research design, inappropriate sample size, or erroneous choice of statistical test for example can all generate misleading results. You are encouraged to be as sceptical and critical about these aspects of empirical research as you are about how the results of research are presented. We will begin with the main culprits you need to know about that can make statistical data misleading. They are:

- measures of central tendency;
- the meaningless 'mean';
- the percentage and proportion;
- relative and absolute risk;
- percentages, proportions, probability and ratios;
- misleading categories;
- failing to look under the lid;
- the correlation that isn't (see Chapter 17);
- when small has a big effect – error of measurement (see Chapter 18);
- extrapolation beyond the reasonable and to the extreme;
- sampling;
- display of data.

All these will now be discussed in more detail.

Measures of central tendency

Let's start with measures of central tendency. As described in Chapter 6, measures of central tendency are measurements used to describe or to give the impression of the 'typical values'. The ways to measure central tendency (common measures of central tendency) are the mean, median and mode. There are many more but we will just discuss these three for now. Deciding which measure of central tendency to use is largely determined by the type of data being collected and analysed when a measure of central tendency is presented it is also normal to include a measure of the variation. One way in which readers can be misled is if an inappropriate measure of central tendency is used to describe a particular sample of data.

An example of this is can be found in relation to income. If you were asked what is the average income for persons in work aged between thirty and thirty-nine in your country, what would you say? For the UK, in 2004/5 the mean value was £26,800. The median however is £20,100 (HMRC 2005), some £6,700 below the mean.

Box 8.1

Why do you think that the discrepancy occurs?

If you wanted to suggest that people were better off than they were then perhaps you would quote the first figure, the mean, but would this be correct? The answer is probably not and certainly not if you quoted this value alone. This is because the distribution of individual incomes does not follow a normal distribution (Chapter 10); it is skewed by those relatively few people who earn a great deal of money, thus the mean is an inappropriate value to quote as a measure of central tendency.

Using the wrong form of central tendency is a common error as well as a way to mislead. Remember to always think about the way the items within a data set are distributed when interpreting your own and other people's statistics.

The meaningless mean

We discussed in Chapter 3 the relationship between the measurement scale and the type of descriptive statistic that should be used when reporting findings. Occasionally you will come across research studies where the wrong type of central tendency has been used. This error is quite often found in relation to numerical data generated through the use of questionnaires.

Let us say, for example, that you have decided to measure patient/client satisfaction in the area in which you work. To save time, you decide to use a questionnaire with one item, this item being a statement 'the service in this area of clinical practice I received was excellent' with options for your patients to express the extent to which they feel that they agree or disagree with this statement. A score of 5 would indicate that they strongly agree, whilst a score of 1 that they strongly disagree. A score of 3 would indicate that they neither agree nor disagree, 2 that they disagree and 4 that they agree. You are rather busy, so you just ask ten patients/clients. Five individuals give your area a score of 2, whilst five give you a score of 4, so how do you report your findings?

Clearly the measurement scale is ordinal, that is the values clearly indicate the direction of the difference (2 is better than 1), but we do not know the magnitude of that difference. The temptation, however, might be to report the arithmetic mean (add up the scores and divide by ten), that is to treat the data as if they were obtained using a ratio measuring scale. If you did this you could report a mean of 3.0, which may look better than confessing that half your clients/patients were not impressed with the service they received.

A more appropriate approach to presenting these data would be to report the percentage of respondents in each category. Often when reporting this type of data we combine the responses from the top two categories and report these as a percentage of the total. Thus in the example above we would say that 50 per cent of the respondents either agreed or strongly agreed with the statement that 'the service in this area of clinical practice I received was excellent'. You would of course need to also state the actual number of respondents.

The percentage and proportion

Percentages are used to express proportions. This is especially important in relation to sample size; for example, we could express the number of people who die from a heart attack in relation to the total number of heart attacks. In the UK the number of people dying from a heart attack was about 10.5 per cent for those admitted to hospital (Chung et al., 2014); initially this statistic looks quite robust, as it is based on a large number of heart attack occurrences. Sometimes percentages are used in situations where the sample size is quite low. In a recent survey we conducted, 80 per cent of the people said they preferred to be at work rather than on holiday. How can this be you might ask? Well we only asked five people, so obtaining such an extreme or unusual result should not be that surprising. The lesson here is to be wary when a **percentage** is quoted without an indication of the **sample** size.

Relative and absolute risk

The efficacy of therapies and treatments are sometimes presented in terms of absolute or relative risk. These two statistics can be used to report risk but even when the data they are based on is the same they can have values which are very different from each other.

Absolute risk is the actual probability that an event will occur. It could, for instance, be your risk of being involved in a car accident whilst driving a car. Relative risk, on the other hand, is a comparison of the risk experienced by one group as compared to another group of people. So, for example, it could be the risk of male drivers being involved in an accident compared to female drivers.

The impacts of health interventions or adjustments in lifestyle are often reported in terms of relative risk. For example, the absolute risk of dying from major heart disease for a person living in England and Wales is approximately 25 per cent or 1:4; in other words, one out of four people is likely to die from major heart disease (ONS, 2011).

The *Daily Mail* newspaper reported a study published in Australia estimating that an individual who spent an hour watching television per day increased their chances of dying through heart failure by 18 per cent, but what does this actually mean in relation to your risk of dying of a heart attack? In fact it increases your overall absolute risk of dying from a heart attack by 4.5 per cent from 25 per cent to 29.5 per cent. Whether this shocks you or not will depend on your own disposition, but it is obvious that a value of 4.5 per cent is less headline grabbing than the relative risk of 18 per cent. Take care when a study records changes in risk that you are aware of the level of the original risk.

The other aspect of the study from Australia, which the researchers certainly alluded to, is that it is not the television per se which is bad for your heart, it's just that the amount of TV that you watch is an indirect measure of how active your lifestyle is.

Percentages, proportions, probability and ratios

It may seem a little strange including quite so many terms in one subheading but they are all related by the fact they can be used to describe risk and are mathematically very similar. In health care situations, percentages, proportions, probability and ratios are often used to describe risk and the chance of benefit from particular interventions.

These measures are not often used to deliberately mislead; however it has been found that humans are not particularly good at transferring risk expressed in terms of probability into a real life context. Many people for instance are disappointed when, having bought a ticket, they do not win the national lottery, and this is despite knowing the actual probability of winning such events is very small indeed. Similarly, you probably know friends, patients or clients who, despite knowing the risks, engage in risky behaviours, seemingly believing that it could not happen to them.

Percentages, proportions and ratios are related mathematical terms. Proportion refers to the number of items in a sub-category in relation to the total amount of the items in the main category, for example the number of men who visited their GP in relation to the total number of people who visited. There are different ways this value could be expressed. For example, we could express the value in terms of the actual data gathered – of 1,223 people who visited the GP in a month 403 were men; as a fraction – roughly 1/3 of those that visited the GP over a period of a month were men; as a decimal – 0.33; as a ratio – 1:2 (ratio of visits by men in relation to other patients); or even as a percentage – 33 per cent. The interesting question is whether or not you instinctively interpret each of these values in a similar way.

Probability

Probability is a measure of chance or risk and is a term that is used extensively in this book. Interestingly we often talk about probability in terms of percentages; for instance there is a 10 per cent chance of an in-patient of an acute hospital obtaining a hospital-acquired infection (HAI). Occasionally this might be expressed as a fraction, i.e. one in ten people admitted to an acute hospital will probably acquire an HAI. Officially, however, probability should be expressed as a decimal with a value between 0 (no chance of an event happening) to 1.0 (certainty).

Box 8.2

Using the example described what is the probability (expressed as a decimal) of getting a HAI).

Given the various ways in which probability can be expressed it is probably no surprise that it has plenty of potential to confuse, particularly given what was described above in relation to human nature and probability. The example below illustrates this a bit further.

Let us say that you are counselling a client about making a choice of contraception. Comparing with a client several forms of contraception, they do not want to use over-intrusive or chemical methods and are considering using a device known as PERSONA (www.persona.info/uk/faq.php) and traditional condoms. The reliability of the PERSONA is given as 94 per cent, whilst that of condoms is considered to be 98 per cent; on the face of it, there does not seem to be much difference.

The reliability of contraceptive methods tends to be compared by looking at how often the method fails over the period of a year and then expressing this value in terms of effectiveness per

100 women over a year. Thus, as male condoms (when used properly) are considered to be 98 per cent effective, what this actually means is that two out of 100 women who use condoms (as the sole means of contraception for a year) will become accidentally pregnant. With respect to the PERSONA device this value is six out of 100. If we compare the efficacy of the two methods it is possible to see that condoms are about three times as effective as the PERSONA device at preventing accidental pregnancies. It is vital to note that both the manufacturers of the PERSONA and of condoms use the standard approved method to describe the risk of pregnancy associated with each approach, and there is certainly no intention to deceive.

Box 8.3

Based on the evidence above, which method of contraception would you recommend to your patient/client?

Another interesting example is given by Darrell Huff, who wrote the seminal book *How to Lie with Statistics*, first published in 1954. Huff (1973) tells us that prior to the introduction of the polio vaccine, the occurrence of polio was reported as being much higher than normal. However, this increased incidence could be largely attributed to an increase in the number of children in the population. Thus, whilst the incidence was high, the actual rate was not significantly different than in previous years. For the health authorities, however, who were trying to persuade as many people as possible to take the new vaccines, it would be extremely convenient for them if they could tell the public that the incidence of polio had apparently increased.

Box 8.4

If you were the US health authorities introducing a vaccine to combat a debilitating disease such as polio, what would you tell the public about the occurrence of polio?

Slight of category

Some data is categorical in nature (see Chapter 3). Subsuming sub-categories within larger categories can be a convenient way to hide detail that you do not want people to see. This type of erroneous presentation is relatively common.

An example of this can often be seen in debates in relation to numbers of employees within the health workforce. In 2012 a UK health minister in the coalition government claimed that despite a period of prolonged austerity the number of qualified clinical practitioners had increased. This in fact was true; however, the number of staff qualified at professional level (i.e. having a qualification recognized by an external regulating professional body, such as occupational therapists and registered nurses) had actually fallen. Was this minister trying to deceive or was he telling the truth? Either way, it is clear that in quoting just an overall figure a substantial variation in the trend in the clinical workforce was being hidden by the answer and more light could have been shed on the issues if trends in the sub-categories of workers had also been reported.

Failing to look under the lid

People are complex. We are different from each other and respond in different ways to the environments that we work and live in. Inevitably, this means that much of the statistical data that we collect will require a complex analysis in order for us to understand it. Failure to perform this analysis or failure to alert people to this complexity will lead to misunderstanding and could mislead; of course, this could be what you are trying to achieve.

A very good example of this can be found in some of the so-called quality statistics (known as performance metrics) applied to universities and colleges. Performance metrics statistics are often used to compile university and college league tables (albeit by the press such as *The Times Higher Education*). When universities appear near the top of these tables, their leaders are apt to laude and publicize their success, but do they know the complexity behind these tables and why certain universities tend to stay at the top? Or are they happy for us to think that these statistics are reliable measures of the quality of learning and teaching at these establishments.

An example of the complexity that underlies such social statistics can be found if the statistics for employability are examined. Contributing to economic growth, prosperity and producing employable graduates is now seen (by governments at least) as a major reason for the existence of universities and colleges. An obvious measure therefore of the success of universities and colleges should be the extent to which their graduates are employed after they have completed their qualification. Of course we should not just be interested in whether they are employed but whether they are employed in the types of jobs that it requires a graduate to do. In the UK the measure used for 'employability' is the number of undergraduates from a particular university or college that are in a 'graduate job' six months after graduation. It is recognized that this six-month figure is not the best measure, but it is applied equally to all of the higher education establishments in the UK. So where is the problem?

Unfortunately, your ability to obtain a good job does not seem to be linked to the quality of the education establishment that you attended, but to many other factors. There is, for example, a strong relationship between the mean qualification score (UCAS points) on entry to university and the percentage of graduates who obtain a 'graduate job' within six months of qualification (Figure 8.1).

Now it could be that well-qualified undergraduates gravitate towards the best quality universities. However, the fact that some of the variation is explicable by entrance qualification, and other sociological data that is available (such as the social class of those that get particular jobs), suggests that the relationship is more likely to result from the fact that in the UK more wealthy parents tend to have children who perform well at school and the link between social class and access to 'good jobs'.

Other factors that influence a university's graduate's ability to obtain graduate employment include institutional reputation, region and locality, the employment market, age profile of the institutions and subject mix (Gibbs 2010). Once these factors are taken into account there is in fact little left that can be attributed to the quality of the institution.

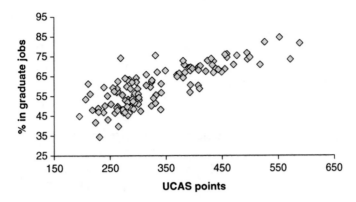

FIGURE 8.1 Plot of the entry qualifications (as measured by UCAS tariff) of students entering UK higher education institutions against the % of UK graduates in jobs that require a degree, 6 months after graduation for the year 2012/13

This example illustrates how complex some analyses need to be to get a full understanding of the data and what it indicates. Faced with a figure that suggests your institution is 'the best' at getting graduates into 'good jobs' how tempting it must be to shout about it, even if you suspect that it has little to do with your institution's actions.

The correlation that isn't

Correlating variables is a common statistical procedure (Chapter 17) used to determine whether one variable is associated with another. That is, if one of the variables changes does the other change also? For example there is a **correlation** between an individual's extent of exposure to passive smoking and their chance of developing lung disease, so we would say that these variables are correlated. However, we cannot infer that two variables are causally linked just because they are correlated. Without more evidence, for instance, we would not be able to say that passive smoking is a cause of lung disease, even though they are correlated.

When small has a big effect – error of measurement

If you are comparing two different groups where the difference between the two groups is potentially small then you need to make sure that your measurement tool is accurate and that the error generated by the measuring tool does not swamp the difference between the two groups. A good example of what can happen when measurement error is not considered relevant was played out by the world's media during the US presidential election between George W. Bush and Al Gore. It was a very closely fought election and everything depended on the way the vote went in the state of Florida. Now you would have thought that ballot papers could be counted without error; unfortunately this is not the case, as humans make errors and, in this case, Florida had used machines to count votes that also generated errors. Unfortunately the size of the errors was larger than the difference in the vote count between Gore and Bush. Each time the votes were recounted a different result was achieved. Several court cases later it was decided that Bush had won; although no one really knows if this was indeed the correct vote. The lesson here is that you should always try to make an estimation of measurement error and when you read studies look to see if it is a relevant consideration.

Extrapolation beyond the reasonable and to the extreme

Sometimes we look particularly at trends in data because we want to make predictions. These predictions are important because they allow us to plan for the future. For example, the trend in increasing obesity in Western countries may allow us to predict the likely future occurrence of type 2 diabetes and thus facilitate the planning of suitable health services. The name for this type of prediction is extrapolation. In extrapolation we predict beyond the current data set. Extrapolations therefore always have an element of unreliability.

An interesting example of this was seen in relation to the Swine Flu (H1N1) pandemic that spread across the world in 2009/10. The 2009/2010 H1N1 flu was a mix of bird, swine and human flu virus. Prior data of such viruses suggested that H1N1 could be a very harmful virus. As a result flu vaccination programmes were widely implemented and anti-viral drugs such as Tamiflu (oseltamivir phosphate) were stockpiled at great cost to national governments.

It turned out that the virus had relatively normal transmissibility for a flu virus, but had low virulence and its mortality was lower than many other previous flu viruses (Wang and Palese 2009) as a result the many government agencies were accused of scaremongering.

You may consider that the extrapolation and actions that governments made in relation to the H1N1 virus were appropriate; after all the first responsibility of governments is to protect citizens. It is, however, a good example of what can happen when an extrapolation is not then reflected in reality. Beware of extrapolations particularly if they seem to go beyond what is reasonable.

Sampling

Problems with sampling are the most likely source of errors within quantitative studies; in most studies these are genuine mistakes and when you review evidence you must pay careful attention to the nature of the sample and whether it was representative of the population being studied. Poor sampling (meaning the sample size or sampling technique does not accurately reflect the population being studied) or lack of appreciation of sampling errors (age, gender, location, size, time-frame) can also generate significant misinterpretation and in some cases deception.

Biased sampling process

The problem of poor sampling technique is illustrated well by a political poll that was taken during the 1948 US presidential election between Thomas Dewey and Harry S. Truman. On the morning after the 1948 presidential election, the *Chicago Daily Tribune*'s headline was 'Dewey

Defeats Truman'. In fact, most of the political reporters and media in the US seemed to believe that Dewey would win; this supposition was built largely on political polls. Unfortunately these polls had in-built biases. Interviewers were given quotas of different types of people such as young, old, male, female and low or high status, but they were given free rein to choose within that sample. This resulted in a biased sample, one that did not represent the whole population. On 2 November 1948, the electorate actually returned Truman as president.

Since these events, pollsters have modified their approaches but still do sometimes predict the results incorrectly. One method that proved remarkably accurate during the 2012 US presidential election was combining the polls taken across the nation using statistical methods devised by Drew Linzer. Drew Linzer not only combines different polls (meta-analysis) but also includes historical trends. Most pollsters during this election said that the election was too close to call. Drew Linzer suggested that it would be Obama, 332 votes, Romney 206, which was how the result turned out (http://votamatic.org). The technique that Linzer uses is based on the premise that individual polls always contain sample bias, but when they are put together in sensible ways they generate reliable results. This premise is also the basis of the meta-analyses that are often used as part of systematic reviews of health research.

The Truman election poll errors highlight some of the issues associated with interviewer bias. Huff (1973) reports a study conducted in the US by the National Opinion Research Center (NORC) during the Second World War where two groups of interviewers were directed to ask a set of questions to 500 African Americans. One group of interviewers was white whilst the other was African American. The questions were overtly controversial and concerned the status of African Americans. One question, for instance, was 'Would Negroes (African Americans) be treated better or worse here if the Japanese conquered the USA?' The African American interviews reported that 9 per cent of their respondents felt life would be better under the Japanese, but this figure dropped to just 2 per cent where the interviewer was white. Responses to other questions confirmed that there was bias being generated through the ethnic background of the interviewer. Unfortunately, Huff (1973) does not give the original reference for this work, but NORC is a highly respected research organization, based at the University of Chicago. Huff's example illustrates how survey data can be subject to biases, which we may not initially consider significant.

Cherry picking and the problem of too small a sample size

Whilst unwittingly introducing sampling bias into a study constitutes a mistake, cherry picking, or deliberately selecting only the data sources that substantiate your view until you get the sample that you want, or omitting to report the results that do not lead to the desired result, is clearly wrong and often represents a more deliberate attempt to deceive. Sometimes cherry picking can occur inadvertently and we may not know that it has happened; such a problem often emerges when the sample size is too small.

Sample size

Let us say, for example, that you are testing a new type of cream for its ability to alleviate dry skin. You apply the cream or a placebo to twenty participants in your work and maybe a few hours after you use some form of objective measure to determine the dryness level of the skin. It turns out that a significant number of individuals in the treatment group report a positive increase in skin hydration relative to the control group. You stop there feeling very happy with the new treatment. Ten days later you notice that someone else has published results on this product, but although they followed the same protocol as you they ended up with no difference between the control and the treatment groups. What has happened?

Unfortunately, your first study fell foul of not having a sufficiently large sample and although you had attempted to obtain a random and representative sample the small sample size used meant that there was a high chance that your sample would not be representative of the whole population. The alternative study, which found no difference, also suffers from the same problem. The solution is to combine the results of the two studies and probably to collect more data.

Take care when considering any study where the sample size is relatively small; a statistical test called a power test can be used to investigate the required sample size for a particular measure.

Ignoring some of the data

A famous advert for a brand of cat food sold in the UK once claimed that eight of ten cats preferred its product. Casting aside the issue that we did not really know what the brand was being tested against, was this claim really credible? When challenged the company could not in fact produce data to show the validity of the results, and were forced to change the claim to eight out of ten owners *who expressed a preference* said their cat preferred it. Presumably many of the owners actually had no preference at all. Of course the company could have told us the percentage of people that really were not bothered as to which cat food they used, but they didn't; instead these apparently less discerning people were simply dropped from the sample. So, was this honest reporting or an attempt to mislead?

A more serious and significant potential example of this type of practice can be found in accusations that have been made concerning current practice within the pharmaceutical industry. Many academic and medical researchers believe that some pharmaceutical industries deliberately withhold data or, at the very least, do not publish all the data appertaining to drug trials that have been performed. Ben Goldacre in his newspaper column refers to this as the problem of 'missing data' (www.badscience.net/). Goldacre (2013) highlights the issue of Tamiflu. Tamiflu is a trade name for the drug oseltamivir phosphate made by the drug company Roche. The UK government spent over 500 million pounds stockpiling Tamiflu in preparation for the 2009/2010 H1N1 flu pandemic. Roche, however, is still considered by many to be withholding data from the Cochrane systematic review of the drugs efficacy.

Box 8.5

Whilst this knowledge does not in itself suggest that Tamiflu is not as effective as claimed, it does cast some doubt. What reasons do you think that Roche might have for not publishing all the information from the trials?

How graphs can be used to persuade

Commonly, data is displayed in graphical form to aid with its interpretation. Unfortunately, graphical representations can also help those who want to persuade rather than inform. Possibly the best-known example of such practice relates to a graph that was placed on the front cover of the 1999 report from the World Meteorological Organization. The graph presented information about changes in global temperature over during the past millennium, highlighting the increase in temperature over the last decade.

The graph was largely based on analyses of 'proxy' records like ice cores, lake sediments and tree ring data. The measurements suggest that temperatures declined in the middle of the millennium and then rose in the first half of the twentieth century. The tree ring data, however, in contrast to both other proxy measures and direct measures (thermometer), imply a decline in temperatures during the twentieth century. The research group that produced the graph decided that the tree ring data during the period when temperatures were increasing was spurious and so they removed these 'indirect' measures from their graph and used direct thermometer readings instead. This meant that the graph was actually based on different types of measurement, which made the increase in global warming appear more smooth and unequivocal than it actually was. The graph was actually used only on the front cover of a document, but was clearly there to have a visual impact rather than to provide accurate information.

The impact of the discovery of this manipulation has become known as 'climategate' and despite the exoneration by various investigations of the scientist involved, it has done lasting damage to the campaigns of those who wish to see stronger governmental action in response to climate change.

Manipulating the axis

Using inappropriate axes for graphs is another way to produce diagrams that have the potential to mislead. Say, for instance, that a trial is run on a novel drug with a potential to relieve

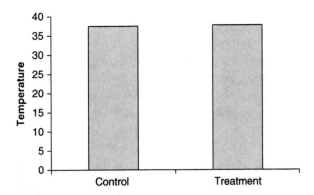

FIGURE 8.2 A hypothetical plot of an experiment with two groups; control and treatment with temperature as the dependent variable. Notice how starting the x-axis at zero reduces the appearance of the difference between the two groups

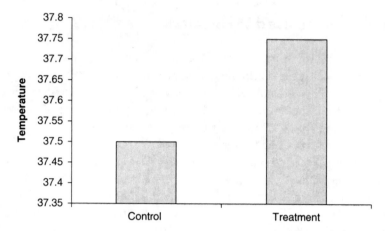

FIGURE 8.3   Depiction of the body temperature of participants from a hypothetical drug trial; note how the graph has been shown such that the difference between treatment and control is emphasized

the pain of arthritis. During the trial some researchers report contra-indications that some participants in the trial seem to have slightly elevated body temperatures. Some follow-up work is undertaken and the results seem to confirm that the drug induces slight pyrexia (mean = 0.25°C), relative to the control group. The company running the trial decides that it needs to show this result but does not want to draw too much attention to it; a bar graph is provided showing the mean body of the control group relative to the test group (Figure 8.2). Notice how, because the y-axis of the graph has been started so low, the difference between the two results appears very small.

If, however, the graph was drawn with the y-axis starting at or just below the normal possible range of human body temperature, say 35°C, this would put more emphasis on the difference between the control and the test group. Given that normal human body temperature fluctuates very little, starting the axis at 35°C is more appropriate (Figure 8.3).

Pictures that perplex

Pictorial diagrams are not used commonly in research papers, but are seen more often in documents such as government reports. Sometimes a picture of a phenomenon is used as part of the overall graphical representation. For example, Figure 8.4 shows the amount of money spent on pharmaceuticals to treat diabetes by the NHS in 2005 and 2010. The height of the medicine bottle represents the amount of spend as measured against the x-axis; note how much larger the bottle for 2010 appears relative to that for 2005.

The actual increase in the bill was 41 per cent, but a quick glance would suggest much more because although the height of the bottle increases in direct proportion to the spending on pharmaceuticals the area of the bottles increases by the square of increase in height. If you come across this style of graph take great care interpreting it and always check that you know the numerical values that underpin the graphical representations.

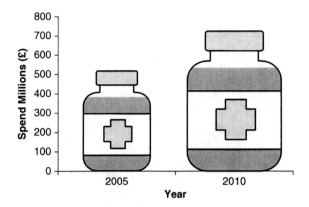

FIGURE 8.4 A plot depicting the change in spend on drugs used to treat diabetes in the UK. Notice how the use of a shape that increases in two dimensions, when the scale (money) increases only in one dimension, gives the visual impression that the increase is greater than it actually is

Having read this chapter and completed the exercises you should be familiar with the following ideas and concepts:

- Not all people use statistics as a means to inform.
- There are numerous ways in which statistics can be used to deceive.
- Errors in the way research is conducted can lead to the production of misleading statistics.

Always read statistical information in a questioning and sceptical way.

9

An introduction to hypothesis testing

Areas of learning covered in this chapter

- What are hypotheses and how are they used in statistics?
- How are hypotheses built?
- What type of errors are there in quantitative studies?
- What is the difference between statistical and clinical significance?

Hypotheses

We will now discuss the concept of hypotheses as they are central to most studies that involve the collection of quantitative data and statistics. But what are hypotheses and more importantly how do they relate to the study of health? Hypotheses are essentially about prediction, which is discussed more fully in Chapter 10. Hypotheses are central to experimental research. Strictly speaking an experiment is an investigation where the researcher controls for some of the variables whilst manipulating others.

When we talk about **hypothesizing** we mean a method of synthesizing an idea or an explanation. A hypothesis is more than simply the idea or theory we are studying. The hypothesis is a proposed explanation for an observation that leads to a prediction(s), that through our investigation and use of statistics we will seek to either confirm or reject and in so doing test the validity of the hypothesis. Hypotheses are generally built from a previous observation or experience.

In general, a hypothesis will lead to a prediction that there is a relationship or link between two or more variables. In investigation (a), described in Chapter 5, we are interested in studying the relationships between sexual activity and sexual health. In investigation (b), we are interested in obesity and how it affects post-operative

> Something to remember:
>
> *hypotheses* is the plural of *hypothesis*.

recovery time. Within these broad areas of study, we have some specific relationships we wish to explore.

Forming the hypothesis for the experiment/study.

One of the hypotheses from investigation (a) is that *males are less likely to use the walk-in clinic than females.* One of the hypotheses from study (b) is that *obese patients treated with Symphadiol will lose weight faster than those not given the drug* (Symphadiol is an entirely fictitious drug). The predictions are highlighted in italics.

Experimental approaches

Some investigations will seek to test these relationships using experiments as a method of finding answers. Experiments attempt to keep the variables we are not interested in constant. This means, for example, in investigation (b), we would split the patients into two groups and subject one group to treatment with Symphadiol.

Box 9.1   Hypothesis building

Observation: A walk-in-clinic manager reports that patients from certain postcode areas seem to be infrequent visitors to the clinic.

Hypothesis: Individuals who live further away from the clinic are less likely to visit.

Experiment/Study: Make a detailed analysis of the distance people live away from the clinic and the frequency of visits.

We could control variables that we were not interested in, such as the patient's sex, age and socio-economic group, by carefully making sure the composition of the two groups was similar. Because we have manipulated one of the groups of people taking part in the study, this investigation is an experiment. Note that in the past people taking part in a study were known as subjects; it is now becoming more common to refer to these people as participants, in recognition that in most cases we must obtain consent from people before we study them and they are therefore participants in the research.

The manipulated group is known as the **experimental group** or **treatment group**; the group not subject to the manipulation is known as the **control group**. Quite often in medical-type studies the control group may receive a placebo, which looks and feels to the participant like the treatment, but has no biological activity. In statistical terms, the experimental treatment and the control groups together are known as the treatment groups. The results of the experiment will be subjected to statistical analysis in order to assess the likelihood of the results occurring by chance.

Non-experimental methods (sometimes called quasi experiments)

The hypotheses from investigation (a) that males are less likely to visit the walk-in clinic than females would probably not use an experiment as the basis for the investigation but a study based on the statistical analysis of data relating to the frequency of visits by males and females. This study would seek to test whether the observed ratio of males to females visiting the clinic was likely to occur by chance. In this type of approach there is no control.

In non-experimental studies rather than control variables we tend to measure all the variables we think could have an influence on the phenomenon of interest. We then try to take account of these variables using statistics. For more guidance on this type of quantitative research design see Depoy and Gitlin (1993).

Having read this section you should now be aware of:

- what is meant by the term hypothesis;
- the difference between an experimental and a non-experimental study;
- by reading Chapter 2 in conjunction with Chapter 9, an understanding of how statistics could be used to test hypotheses.

Variables

Given that we have determined that a hypothesis is a prediction concerning two or more variables, it is important that we remain aware of the role of each of the variables when we apply a statistical test. For the statistical tests described in this book, we will have one **dependent variable** and at least one **independent variable**.

Dependent variable

As the name implies, the dependent variable refers to a variable whose value is determined or dependent on the value of another variable. We may, for example, hypothesize that blood pressure and age are linked. If we were studying this relationship the dependent variable would be blood pressure, as we would be predicting that age in some way was important in determining blood pressure. We could not, however, suggest that age was determined by blood pressure.

Independent variable

The independent variable, on the other hand, is the one thought by the researcher to determine the value (at least in part) of the dependent variable. If we consider the relationship between blood pressure and age, we could suggest that age in some way may account for the level of blood pressure recorded; thus age is the independent variable. For experimental designs, the independent variable is the variable that is fixed or manipulated by the person doing the experiment. If looking, for example, at the relationship between bacterial growth in culture and temperature, the experimenters control the range of temperatures they wish to use. In experimental designs, the independent variable is always the variable that is manipulated.

In the experiment described above the independent variable is the treatment group (either Symphadiol treated or control) the patients are assigned to, while the dependent variable is the weight loss. Weight loss is the variable that will be measured.

In the study of visits to the walk-in-clinic and distance travelled, distance travelled will be the independent variable, and number of visits to the clinic the dependent variable. This is so because we are hypothesizing that the number of visits to the walk-in-clinic will depend on how close the patient lives to the clinic.

Other variables

Another important type of variable is the **confounding variable**.

A confounding variable is one that has influence on the value of the dependent variable yet it is not important with respect to the hypothesis that is being tested. For example, in the test of the impact of Symphadiol, it could be that *age* of the patient *influences* the effects of Symphadiol. If this is the case and we fail to ensure that both treatment groups have participants of similar age then age will become a confounding variable, and the results of our experiment may be difficult to interpret. Potential confounding variables need to be taken into account using appropriate and carefully thought out research designs particularly with respect to the selection of the sample.

Box 9.3   Short exercise

Find two research papers on a subject that interests you where the authors have used statistics. For each study, decide:

1. What the hypothesis is.
2. How many variables are being tested.
3. What the independent variable(s) is.
4. What the dependent variable(s) is.
5. How many treatment groups there are.

Errors and statistics

In statistical terms an error is something that may give us a false result. There are several types of error. They fall into four categories: random error, sampling error, measurement error and experimental error, discussed at length in Chapter 3. Much of research design and statistics involves either trying to reduce error or trying to take account of it. One of the most important uses of statistics is thus to help decide if an observed result could be due to chance, i.e. caused by sampling and other non-systematic errors.

Let's say that you are carrying out the investigation on symphadiol (b). Having collected the data (Chapter 5), plotted and calculated the means you will see that there is a difference between the group of patients that were treated with Symphadiol and those that were not. The question facing the researcher analysing the data is: is this difference due to **chance** or is it due to the **treatment?** Such questions form the basis of all statistical testing.

Box 9.4 Chance

By chance, we mean something that just happens by luck or fortuitously, something without an assignable cause. Random is another name for an event determined by chance.

We no longer just want to describe the data; we want to use statistics to infer things from our data and enhance the treatment and care of patients. So the important question for the researcher is: are the relationships we see down to chance? On the other hand, are they real? Errors can lead us to make incorrect conclusions. The use of statistics will help inform us if the observed result is valid (meaning real) or if it is caused by chance.

The statistical hypothesis

The researcher establishes an experimental hypothesis before performing an experiment or study to test it. In a similar fashion, when we test the results of the experiment to see if they could have occurred by chance, we also establish a statistical hypothesis. The most common form of statistical hypothesis found is the hypothesis of no difference, often called the **null hypothesis** and given the symbol H_o.

It is here that beginners at statistics often become a little confused. Take your time and practise using the exercises supplied.

Observation

In the study of the walk-in centre, we would gather data on frequency of visit by males and females to the centre. Having displayed these data in an appropriate manner we notice there is a difference in the frequency of visits of males and females: this is known as the observation.

Null hypothesis

The null hypothesis for this observation is that although there appears to be a difference in the frequency of visits between males and females this observation is caused by chance and in an investigation based on the whole population there would *not* be a difference.

We would now conduct a statistical test that is appropriate (i.e. a test design for the type of data that was collected); the answer to this test would give us an indication of the probability of the observation being due to chance. From this test we would either reject or accept the null hypothesis.

In the study of the effects of Symphadiol on weight loss, we would gather data on the weight loss of the groups of patients, those who were given the drug and the others who were not. Having completed the study and plotted the data using a bar chart (see Chapter 7) you can see that there is a difference between the treatment groups.

The null hypothesis for this observation is that although there appears to be a difference between the two treatment groups (i.e. the group of participants given the drug showed greater weight loss than those who didn't), this observation is caused by chance and in an investigation based on the whole population there would *not* be a difference between the two variables.

We would now conduct a statistical test that is appropriate; the answer to this test would give us an indication of the probability of the observation being due to chance. From this test we would either reject or accept the null hypothesis.

If we reject the null hypothesis, we then say that the observed observation is **statistically significant**. This is a very important concept and means that we have a certain degree of certainty that the observed result is real and would be reflected in the whole population.

As well as the null hypothesis you may also find that some textbooks refer to the alternative hypothesis, given the symbol H_1. As the name implies this is the opposite of the null hypothesis and a source of confusion amongst new researchers. If the H_0 (null) hypothesis is that there is no difference between treatment groups then the alternative is that there is a difference. When learning statistics it is best to stick with thinking about the null hypothesis; this helps avoiding addled brains.

In research papers, it is common to find that the statistical hypotheses are implied rather than stated explicitly. Again, it is a good idea, until you become confident with statistics, to state what the null hypothesis is before conducting a statistical test.

Types of interaction between variables

When we conduct studies, we are not always looking for the same type of relationship between variables. In general, there are three types of interaction: *differences*, relationships and *associations*.

Deciding on the type of interaction between the variables you are dealing with is a very important aspect of statistics. This is because the type of interaction between variables will in part determine the statistical test that you use.

What is meant by difference is clear cut. In the Symphadiol experiment we were looking to see if there was a *difference* in the weight loss between the treatment groups. If we are looking for a relationship we would be looking to see if two (or more) variables vary with each other; i.e. if you change one variable, do you get a change in the other? For example, is the incidence of lung cancer related to the number of cigarettes smoked each day?

In the walk-in clinic study, we were looking to see if there was an *association* between gender and frequency of visit. An association is really a special form of relationship but here we were asking the question: is one variable commonly found with a second variable? For example, we could ask the question: is skin cancer found more commonly (associated) in males or females?

The problem with clinical and statistical significance

Just because you find a result isn't caused by chance (statistically significant) doesn't mean you paint the town red or even jump out of the bath shouting 'Eureka!' Now is the time for some calm thinking. Was your experiment or study conducted correctly? When research papers are published or sent for review the authors will always say their results are significant but the critics will always question whether or not the experiment was conducted correctly. Statistics cannot make up for poor experimental design.

Just because a result is statistically significant doesn't mean it is of clinical significance, i.e. that practice should be altered because of it. Let's imagine that you discover that drinking three pints of water per day reduces the incidence of acute myeloid leukemia (AML) by 10 per cent. In other words one in ten people who previously would have contracted AML will no longer do so, as long as everyone drinks three pints of water per day. If, however the incidence of contracting AML is just 1/32,500, drinking three pints of water will reduce this to just 1/35,750. Is this a sufficient drop to justify the recommendation?

In health care it is also essential that we take into account any side effects of proposed treatments. Would the reduction in incidence of AML justify all those extra visits to the toilet?

1. For the study on Symphadiol explained in Chapter 5, if you were just looking at the effect of Symphadiol (not exercise) describe: (a) the experimental hypothesis (if one exists); (b) the statistical hypothesis (H_1); (c) the null hypothesis H_0; (d) the independent variable; (e) the dependent variable.
2. For each of the experiments/studies given in Chapter 5 describe the likely source of error.

Having read this chapter and completed the exercises, you should be familiar with the follow ideas and words:

- experimental and statistical hypothesis;
- control group;
- experimental treatment group;
- treatment groups;
- statistically significant;
- in statistical terms what is meant by difference, association and relationship;
- the difference between statistical and clinical significance;
- independent, dependent and confounding variables;
- chance;
- error.

10

Distributions and probabilities

Areas of learning covered in this chapter

- What are probabilities?
- How are probabilities linked to statistic and frequency distributions?
- How can frequency distributions be used to make predictions?
- What types of distributions are there?

One of the more important concepts in statistics is the idea that numbers can be distributed in certain ways. What we mean by distributed is the frequency of occurrence of particular numbers. For example, a data set of the number of sexual partners each individual has during a lifetime could contain just the values 4 or 3, though it's much more likely that it will be a mixture of different numbers from higher to lower. The mixture is very important, largely because the way your numbers are mixed or distributed will determine the type of statistical test that you use. The easiest way to see the way in which data combinations are assembled is to plot them in a frequency **histogram**.

Frequency histograms

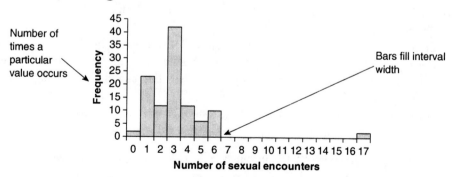

FIGURE 10.1 A histogram showing the frequency distribution of number of sexual partners for 109 women aged thirty, who responded to a questionnaire distributed in the Southwark district of London UK

The frequency histogram is really a type of bar chart where the y-axis is the frequency of occurrence of a particular case. On the x-axis, we have a scale that is bounded by the values of the lowest and the highest of the cases. In between are placed the values of the scale using suitable intervals. A bar is drawn that fills the whole of each of the intervals being measured; the sides of the bars are parallel and the width of the bar held constant.

This type of figure is normally used for variables that are recorded on an **interval** or **ratio scale**. If your data is interval or ratio scale, plotting it in this manner must be one of your very first steps. This is because the distributions of data and numbers form the basis of many statistical tests. You will find that numbers can be distributed in many ways. Some of these distributions have characteristics that can be exploited by researchers. One such distribution that we shall go on to explore is the **normal distribution**. This distribution forms the basis of many statistical tests, but first we need to discuss **probability**.

> Using the data given in Chapter 5 for the walk-in clinic, produce a frequency histogram for the number of sexual encounters reported during a three-month period.

Probability and statistics

In Chapter 9 we introduced the notion of a statistical test and discussed the idea that we perform statistical tests because we want to know whether the results we obtain are due to the experimental treatment or to chance. Chance is a word that has the same meaning as the word probability. When we say, 'What is the chance of patient x catching malaria?' we could also say, 'What is the probability?' We could also say, 'What is the likelihood?' These phrases all have the same meaning: we want to know whether something is likely to happen or not. Of these terms, probability is used more by statisticians. It is given the symbol P. P is normally described as values between zero (not possible) and 1 (certainty). The probability that you will die is 1; the probability that you will meet Florence Nightingale is 0.

Often in the media and elsewhere you will see probabilities reported as percentages. In this case, the probability that you will die would be recorded as 100 per cent and of your meeting Florence Nightingale 0 per cent.

To help put probability more into context, imagine that you are walking down a busy street on a weekend with your eyes closed (do not try this at home), then you suddenly open your eyes. The probability of seeing a man will be 0.5 or 50 per cent. The probability of seeing a woman will also be 0.5 (or half of 100%).

What does this probability mean? Half the time when you open your eyes you will see a woman and the other half a man. How do we get from a value of 0.5 to a more meaningful fraction?

Well 0.5 can also be written as $\frac{0.5}{1}$ (try putting 0.5 in your calculator and dividing it by 1) $\frac{0.5}{1}$ is the same as $\frac{1}{2}$ (try putting 1 in your calculator and dividing it by 2). In statistics we record a probability of $\frac{1}{2}$ as P = 0.5. In statistical testing we need to be at least 95 per cent certain that the result we obtained is true (i.e. not caused by sampling error). In statistics, however, we normally express this probability in terms of doubt; thus rather than say we want to be 95 per cent certain we would say that we are 5 per cent uncertain that the result is true. This 5 per cent value is normally expressed as $P = 0.05$. Remember P stands for probability.

Box 10.1 Expressing probabilities

Probabilities can be expressed as:

1. a value between 0 and 1;
2. a percentage;
3. a fraction.

How are probabilities and distributions linked?

Say you have a bag of laundry with equal numbers of blue and pink towels. You cannot see into the bag. When you reach in and pull out a towel there are two possible outcomes: the towel will be pink or the towel will be blue.

Box 10.2 Practising your maths

1. Express 0.45 as a fraction.
2. Express 0.45 as a percentage.
3. If you walked into a room that was occupied by fifty-five men and forty-five women what is the probability that a woman would be the first person that you encountered?
4. What is $\frac{2}{3}$ expressed as a probability?
5. What is $\frac{2}{5}$ expressed as a percentage?

Now if you pull out two towels the number of possible outcomes increases: it could be two blue towels in a row (BB) or a pink towel twice in a row (PP), or pink and then blue (PB), or blue and then pink (BP). In fact, we have four possible outcomes. So, with just two events the number of outcomes and complexity is increasing. However, we can still predict what the probable combination of pink or blue towels might be.

If there are four outcomes (BB, PP, PB and BP) then the chance that any one of these combinations occurring is 0.25 or $\frac{1}{4}$. Two of these outcomes give you essentially the same combination of towels (PB, BP). Thus the chance of ending up with two pink towels in your hand is $\frac{1}{4}$ and two blue towels $\frac{1}{4}$ and one blue and one pink towel $\frac{1}{2}$ i.e. $\frac{1}{4} + \frac{1}{4}$.

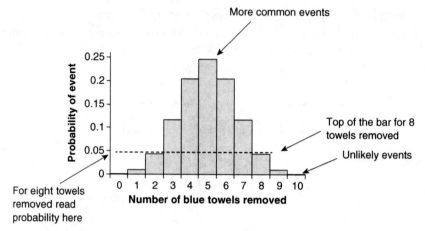

FIGURE 10.2   A histogram showing the probability of removing various combinations of blue and pink towels from a bag consisting of a number of blue and pink towels in equal proportion

Let's work through the obvious next step. You draw out three towels from your bag. The possible outcomes are PPP, BBB, PBB, BBP, PPB, BPP, BPB and PBP – there are eight of them. The probability of each outcome occurring is thus $\frac{1}{8}$. We have four combinations, all blue or all pink, or one pink and two blue, or two blue and one pink. So, what is the probability of obtaining each of these combinations? For PPP and BBB it is straightforward as we have already said the probability of these outcomes is $\frac{1}{8}$. There are three outcomes that give us one pink and two blue towels, so the probability of this combination is $\frac{1}{8} + \frac{1}{8} + \frac{1}{8} = \frac{3}{8}$. There are also three outcomes that give us one blue and two pink towels, so the probability of this combination is $\frac{1}{8} + \frac{1}{8} + \frac{1}{8} = \frac{3}{8}$.

I'm sure you can see that as the number of events increases so the probability of each of the outcomes changes. As the events increase, we need to use graphics (see Figure 10.2). It is possible to draw a histogram that shows the probability of obtaining certain combinations given a certain number of events. Let's say you were pulling out 10 of the towels, now if you work through the maths you will find that here there are 11 combinations.

Using Figure 10.2, a frequency histogram, it is possible to say just how unlucky you had been, if whilst searching for ten pink towels you actually pulled out eight blue towels. (Find eight blue towels on the *x*-axis, go up to the top of the bar and read off the value on the *y*-axis.)

Box 10.3   Flipping coins

If you flip a coin ten times what is the probability that a head will be turned up just three times? Use Figure 9.2 to help.

The type of distribution shown here (Figure 10.2) is called the **binomial distribution**. We have seen how it can be used to predict how rare or unusual certain events will be. This is the basis of statistical testing – asking the question what is the probability (chance) of obtaining a result by chance? Clearly, in the example above, to pull out ten blue towels represents a rare event. We can also see that distributions of numbers and probabilities are linked.

Now the important thing about certain distributions is that they allow us to make predictions and fortunately it just so happens that many natural phenomena produce data sets that have a distribution that is similar to the one above. This distribution is known as the **normal** or Gaussian distribution. This distribution forms the basis for many of the most commonly used statistics. The type of statistics that rely on numbers being distributed in a certain way are called **parametric statistics**. We will now explore the normal distribution.

Having read this section you should be aware of:

- what is meant by the term probability and the ways in which probabilities can be expressed;
- that it is possible using a knowledge of how numbers are distributed to make predictions.

The normal distribution curve

Imagine that the intervals on the *x*-axis were infinitely small. Instead of a bar chart with steps we could produce a curve, particularly if we didn't shade in the bars. The normal distribution would look like such a curve. The normal distribution has mathematical properties that allow us to make predictions, just like the histogram above. Note also how it is drawn, in very much the same way as Figure 10.1, as if we had connected the top of the bars with a line and then removed the bars.

As a defined distribution curve of numbers, the normal distribution has certain properties. The first is the very obvious: the curve is symmetrical – you could almost say it had a certain beauty, it is sometimes referred to as bell shaped. The exact shape of the curve will depend on the standard

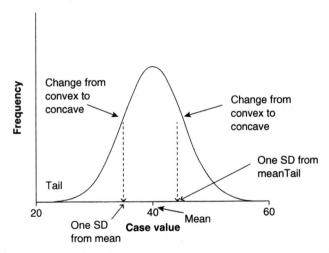

FIGURE 10.3 The normal distribution curve, shown here with a mean of 40 and a standard deviation (SD) of 8

deviation of the data. It's worth remembering that the normal distribution is the construct of a mathematician's mind, so few data sets are likely to give data that exactly match the normal curve.

The tails of a normally distributed curve (the rare values) tend to be short. Nevertheless, probably the most important feature of the normal distribution curve is that at the points where the curve changes from being concave to convex (point of inflection) it is always one standard deviation (SD) away from the mean. The mean is always in the middle of the x-axis. What this tells us is that the area enclosed by the boundaries of the mean plus one standard deviation and the mean minus one standard deviation is always a constant proportion of the total area, namely 68.27 per cent.

If we were to move two standard deviations away from either side of the mean then we would encapsulate 95.44 per cent of the total area. If you were to take a large sample of patients' arm lengths, you would expect that 68.27 per cent of your results would lie within ± 1 SD of the mean and that 95.44 per cent would lie within ± 2 SD of the mean.

Box 10.4   The normal distribution

1. is bell shaped;
2. is symmetrical;
3. has short tails ;
4. has points of inflection that are always 1 SD away from the mean.

In a normally distributed data one standard deviation either side of the mean always encloses 68.72 per cent of the data set.

We have now introduced a method by which if we know the mean and the standard deviation of a set of data and we know that it is normally distributed then we can make predictions. We use this knowledge as the basis of what are often called **parametric statistics**.

Box 10.5   Making a prediction

You are interested in the number of Opsite® dressings used on the average medical ward. You collect data from 102 wards. The data are normally distributed. How many wards will lie within ± 1 SD of the mean?

Hint: in normally distributed data 68.27 per cent of the data lies within ± 1 SD of the mean.

Deviations from the normal distribution

Sometimes we find that the data we have collected does not fit the normal distribution. The best way to get a rough idea if your data fits the distribution is to plot a frequency histogram. Some deviations have a particular shape and are given special names.

The distribution shown in Figure 10.4 is called negatively skewed. This is because the mean lies to the left of the median (as you look at it).

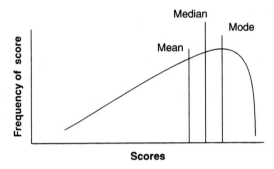

FIGURE 10.4   A negatively skewed distribution

The distribution shown in Figure 10.5 is called positively skewed. This is because the mean lies to the right of the median.

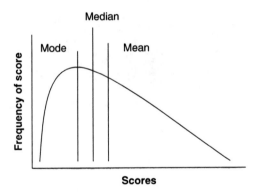

FIGURE 10.5   A positively skewed distribution

Skewed data sets tend to occur when there are values which are much greater or lower than the rest. Thus the frequency histogram is not symmetrical, it's skewed. In these distributions the greater the difference between the mean and the median the greater the skew or skewness.

It is also possible to have symmetrical distributions that do not conform to the normal distribution. The most common to come across are random distributions and the regular or underdispersed distribution examples of which are given below.

Random and clumped distributions

Data sets where the variance is roughly equal to the mean are referred to as *randomly distributed*. Random distribution tends to be uncommon. An example of a random distribution could be the number of occurrences of certain diseases within defined geographical areas. Such a distribution is shown in Figure 10.6 for the disease cystic fibrosis.

It should be noted that true randomness is comparatively uncommon and that the geographical distribution of many disease phenomena tends to be clumped or over-dispersed. We talk of disease outbreaks where we recognize that particular areas have a high incidence of a certain disease. In random phenomena we are saying that each event (an occurrence of cystic fibrosis) in unrelated to any other occurrence. If the distribution is clumped it suggests that the events are related, for example in the case of a contagious disease, or a disease that is triggered by some environmental factor. Clumped distributions tend to show a strong positive skew (mean lies to the right of the median). Such a distribution is shown for the occurrence of AIDS cases across the metropolitan districts of the USA.

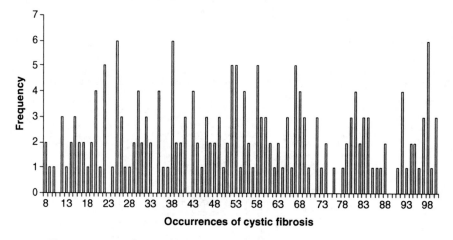

FIGURE 10.6   The occurrence of cystic fibrosis within the UK as recorded by parish

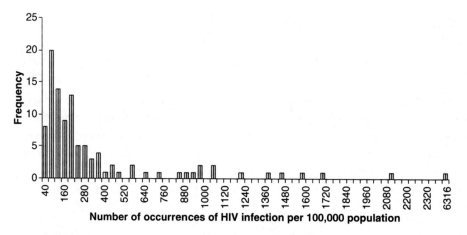

FIGURE 10.7   AIDS cases per 100,000 population, by metropolitan area reported in 1999. Note that the point after the value of 2080 has a value of 6316 and thus the x-axis has been truncated. This distribution shows a strong positive skew, and thus these data are clumped. The mean is 359, median 162 and the mode 47 (www.cdc.gov/hiv/stats/hasrlink.htm)

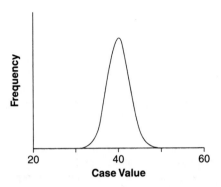

FIGURE 10.8 A regular distribution with a mean of 40 and a standard deviation of 2

The last distribution we want to make you aware of is that of the **regular distribution**. The regular distribution is really an extreme form of the normal distribution. In regular distributions, the standard deviation is small in relation to the mean, that is there is very little spread in the data set. An example of this could be records of the number of fingers and toes within a population. Obviously, people with fewer than twenty fingers and toes are very unusual and so the distribution would be regular. If a normal distribution is shaped like that shown in Figure 10.8 it is said to show **kurtosis**. It can also be said to show kurtosis if the point of the curve is flattened.

It is important that you can distinguish between clumped and random distributions. The manner in which data are distributed is important as they tell us about the fundamental properties we are studying and as we have seen they are very relevant to studies of the distribution and spread of disease (epidemiology). We also need to know how data are distributed before we embark on many statistical tests. We can distinguish between the different types of distribution using statistical tests that will be explained later.

Having read this chapter and completed the exercises, you should be familiar with the follow ideas and words:

- frequency histogram;
- regular distribution;
- probability;
- random and clumped distribution;
- normal distribution;
- skewness and kurtosis;

- the concept of a distribution of numbers and how it links to probability;
- the properties of the normal distribution;
- the importance of knowing how your data are distributed.

1. Collect measurement of the lengths of the index finger from twenty individuals and plot these data using a frequency histogram. Record the sex of your participants. Discuss your result. Which distribution does your figure look like?

(Continued)

EXERCISES

(Continued)

2. Repeat exercise 1, but increase your sample size. If you are working with a group of people you may want to amalgamate your results (but only if you took measurements from different participants). Discuss your result: (a) Which distribution does your figure look like? (b) Has the shape of the distribution changed? What does this tell you? (c) What happens to the distribution if you separate out the male participants from the females?

3. If you tossed a coin four times what are: (a) the potential combination of outcomes; (b) the probability of each outcome? (c) What is the probability if a coin is tossed four times of obtaining three heads and one tail? (d) Plot the frequency distribution of the weight loss of two of the treatment groups from the Symphadiol experiment as they are at the end of the study. Do the distributions tell us anything?

11

Making predictions

This chapter begins with a little reminder. Most health care professionals learn a lot of their art through practice. So it is with statistics; don't expect to become a practitioner of statistics without practice.

Areas of learning covered in this chapter

- How to estimate how close a sample mean is to the population mean.
- What is the standard error?
- How are confidence limits calculated?
- What are z scores and how can they be used to make predictions?

You have seen how we can use statistics to describe data, how data can be presented as distributions of numbers and in theory how a distribution can be used to make predictions. Now we want to show you how these predictions are made. We want to know in this case how unusual a particular event is likely to be.

The first statistic we will describe is a statistic that isn't often thought of as a prediction at all, but it most definitely is. It is also one of the most quoted statistics, and it's called the **standard error of the sample mean** (SE). So, what is it? And why is it often quoted?

The standard error of the mean provides a prediction of how close a **sample mean** is to the true **population mean**. In other words, how good was the sample? As such, it is a vital statistic. Remember we take samples of populations normally because we don't have the resources to collect the data from the whole population. The SE is a prediction that suggests how close our measure (taken from the sample) is to that of the true population.

Central limit theorem and standard error

The standard error relies on a 'statistical law' called the **central limit theorem**. The law basically states that if you were to collect a whole series of samples, and then plot a frequency histogram of the means of those samples, the distribution produced would be normally distributed, with the mean of that distribution (if you had collected enough samples, the samples have to be taken randomly) being the population mean. You may want to try and prove this to yourself (see Box 11.1).

So how does the central limit theorem help us? Well, as this distribution of the means of samples is normal in shape it will have the same inflected shoulders as any other normal distribution. If you remember, if we take a vertical line down to intercept the x-axis, the point at which the interception occurs is normally known as the standard deviation. In the case of the distribution of sample means, it could be known as the 'standard deviation of sample means' but, for simplicity, we call it the **standard error.** Just with the standard deviation, if we take the values that range from 1 SE below to 1 SE above the population mean, we will have 68.27 per cent of all the sample means. We can also predict with 68.27 per cent confidence that the population mean will be within ±1 SE of any sample mean. The standard error is simple to calculate. It is the standard deviation divided by the square route of the sample size, or:

$$SE = \frac{s}{\sqrt{n}}$$

where s is the standard deviation and n is the sample size. When calculating the standard error by hand find the square root of the sample size first.

Box 11.1

Look at the sample of heights of the control participants in the Symphadiol experiment (Chapter 5).

1. The total mean of the heights for the two groups is 179.7, but for each sub-sample it differs. They differ because of sampling error (see Chapter 3). Plot the mean of each sample as a frequency histogram.
2. What shape does your histogram have?

The standard error of the sample mean is a prediction of how accurate a measure your sample mean is in relation to the population mean. Notice the larger the standard deviation the larger the standard error. Remember P is shorthand for *the probability of this is ...*

In the example from Box 11.1 you would have found the mean to be 179.7 ± 1.97. What this tells us is that we can be 68.27 per cent confident that the mean lies somewhere between 179.7 − 1.97 and 179.7 + 1.97, or between 177.7 and 181.7. Of course, what 68.26 per cent confidence means is that in only approximately sixty-eight times out of 100 would this prediction be correct. In statistical terms we would say P = 0.68, or the probability of the population mean lying in this range is 0.68. It stands to reason therefore, that the probability of it not being in that range is 0.32. In other words in approximately thirty-two times out of 100 the prediction would be wrong and the population mean would lie outside of the predicted boundaries.

Box 11.2

Look at the data for heights from the Symphadiol experiment again. Take five cases and calculate the standard error, take ten cases and calculate the SE, and finally take fifteen cases and produce another SE.

- What does this tell you about the relationship between sample size and the SE?
- What would happen to the SE if the variability was lower? (Remember we use the standard deviation as the measure of variability.)
- What is the relationship between variability and the SE?

Note the standard error has meaning only if the data set is normally distributed. The standard error is a parametric statistic.

How to increase your confidence

Now, whilst you may bet £5 on a horse with odds of 68 in 100 of winning the race, it would be foolish to change a health care procedure based on those odds. Really, you would like to have greater confidence in the predictions concerning health care. In practice researchers like to have 95 per cent confidence or above that the result has not occurred by chance. In some medical studies 99 per cent confidence is the accepted level. In reporting the results of statistical test, we normally report the probability of the result occurring by chance. Thus, to have what is known as a statistically significant result P (probability) must be = to 0.05 or less, whilst in some medical studies P must be equal to 0.01 or less.

Calculating confidence limits (this method works only for large samples where N is greater than 30)

If we want to be 95 per cent confident in the boundaries that we predicted for the value of the population mean in relation to our estimate then all we need to do is set the boundaries to our estimate as:

mean ± 1.96 x SE.

If we want to be 99 per cent confident we use the mean ± 2.58 x SE.

Of course, we haven't plucked these values from the air and if you want to know where they have come from you will have to read on.

Example from the literature 11.1   Do nurse-led services reduce duration of stay in acute care units?

The cost of care is important to all health systems. Reducing the amount of time spent in care can deliver savings. There have been many studies of how variation in care delivery can alter the duration of stay. In Griffiths et al.'s (2001) study, the duration of stay was measured in the context of intermediate care delivery, where acute services were substituted for a nursing-led in-patient care unit. The researchers found that under this new regime the duration of stay increased. Table 11.5 in their study shows the mean stay length in traditional and nurse-led units. It gives confidence limits in the last column, for example mean length of stay of 36.9 days with 95 per cent confidence limits of 29.3 to 44.5. This means that the authors are predicting that the population mean lies with the range of 29.3 to 44.5 and they have 95 per cent confidence in that prediction. You can read more of this interesting study at: http://ageing.oxfordjournals.org/content/30/6/483.full.pdf+html.

Z scores

The values we used to calculate the 95 per cent and 99 per cent confidence limits are z scores from the normal distribution.

Once you become more familiar with statistics, you will forget that we use z scores to give confidence limits. However, despite being a forgotten statistic z scores can help us make predictions and plan appropriately.

So, what is a z score?

A **z score** is a measure of the distance along the horizontal (x-axis) of a normal distribution measured in units of standard deviation. This sounds complex but isn't really.

Try to imagine it like this. Say you wanted to compare how much variation there was in the lung volume amongst people of different countries, the only problem being each country used a different set of instruments to measure lung volume, some that measured in litres, some in pints and some in cubic feet. The first thing that you would want to do is to convert all the measurements to one type, a standard.

In statistics, it is exactly the same; if we want to measure how unusual a particular case will be we need to use a standard. We have already discussed one type of standard measurement, the standard deviation. In a normal distribution, the cases that lie between + or – one standard deviation will always make up 68.26 per cent of the entire data set. What is a z score then? It's the distance between the mean and any other value of interest stated in units of standard deviation. A z score of 1 is = to 1 SD. As we have said, move away from the mean in both directions, i.e. + and – by one standard deviation, and you will have enclosed 68.26 per cent of all the cases in your distribution (see Chapter 10). If you move ±2 standard deviations ($z = 2$) away from the mean you will enclose 95.44 per cent of all cases. As it happens ± 1.96 SD ($z = \pm$) encloses 95 per cent of all cases and ± 2.58 SD (±2.58 Z) encloses 99 per cent. Thus, a z score is simply a multiple of SDs.

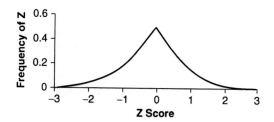

Figure 11.1 Proportion of cases cut off for a given value of *z*

For any given case, we can calculate a *z* score. You calculate a *z* score as

$$z = \frac{\text{case} - \text{mean}}{\text{standard deviation}}$$

$$\text{Or } z = \frac{x - \bar{x}}{S}$$

OK, so what can we do with this *z* score? Making predictions

What a *z* score can tell us is the proportion of cases that will be enclosed between the mean and that score. To find this proportion we would normally use a table of *z* scores, as in Table 11.1.

Table 11.1 Areas of the normal distribution curve as determined by *z* score

z	0	0.01	0.02	0.03	0.04	0.05	0.06	0.07	0.08	0.09
0	0.5	0.496	0.492	0.488	0.484	0.4801	0.4761	0.4721	0.4681	0.4641
0.1	0.4602	0.4562	0.4522	0.4483	0.4443	0.4404	0.4364	0.4325	0.4286	0.4247
0.2	0.4207	0.4168	0.4129	0.409	0.4052	0.4013	0.3974	0.3936	0.3897	0.3859
0.3	0.3821	0.3783	0.3745	0.3707	0.3669	0.3632	0.3594	0.3557	0.352	0.3483
0.4	0.3446	0.3409	0.3372	0.3336	0.33	0.3264	0.3228	0.3192	0.3156	0.3121
0.5	0.3085	0.305	0.3015	0.2981	0.2946	0.2912	0.2877	0.2843	0.281	0.2776
0.6	0.2743	0.2709	0.2676	0.2643	0.2611	0.2578	0.2546	0.2514	0.2483	0.2451
0.7	0.2420	0.2389	0.2358	0.2327	0.2296	**0.2266**	0.2236	0.2206	0.2177	0.2148
0.8	0.2119	0.209	0.2061	0.2033	0.2005	0.1977	0.1949	0.1922	0.1894	0.1867
0.9	0.1841	0.1814	0.1788	0.1762	0.1736	0.1711	0.1685	0.166	0.1635	0.1611
1.0	0.1587	0.1562	0.1539	0.1515	0.1492	0.1469	0.1446	0.1423	0.1401	0.1379
1.1	0.1357	0.1335	0.1314	0.1292	0.1271	0.1251	0.1230	0.1210	0.1190	0.1170
1.2	0.1151	0.1131	0.1112	0.1093	0.1075	0.1056	0.1038	0.1020	0.1003	0.0985
1.3	0.0968	0.0951	0.0934	0.0918	0.0901	0.0885	0.0869	0.0853	0.0838	0.0823

(Continued)

TABLE 11.1   (Continued)

z	O	0.01	0.02	0.03	0.04	0.05	0.06	0.07	0.08	0.09
1.4	0.0808	0.0793	0.0778	0.0764	0.0749	0.0735	0.0721	0.0708	0.0694	0.0681
1.5	0.0668	0.0655	0.0643	0.063	0.0618	0.0606	0.0594	0.0582	0.0571	0.0559
1.6	0.0548	0.0537	0.0526	0.0516	0.0505	0.0495	0.0485	0.0475	0.0465	0.0455
1.7	0.0446	0.0436	0.0427	0.0418	0.0409	0.0401	0.0932	0.0384	0.0375	0.0367
1.8	0.0359	0.0351	0.0344	0.0336	0.0329	0.0322	0.0314	0.0307	0.0301	0.0294
1.9	0.0287	0.0281	0.0274	0.0268	0.0262	0.0256	0.025	0.0244	0.0239	0.0233
2.0	0.0228	0.0222	0.0217	0.0212	0.0207	0.0202	0.0197	0.0192	0.0188	0.0183
2.1	0.0179	0.0174	0.017	0.0166	0.0162	0.0158	0.0154	0.015	0.0146	0.0143
2.2	0.0139	0.0136	0.0132	0.0129	0.0125	0.0122	0.0119	0.0116	0.0113	**0.0110**
2.3	0.0107	0.0104	0.0102	0.0099	0.0096	0.0094	0.0091	0.0089	0.0087	0.0084
2.4	0.0082	0.008	0.0078	0.0075	0.0073	0.0071	0.0069	0.0068	0.0066	0.0064
2.5	0.0062	0.006	0.0059	0.0057	0.0055	0.0054	0.0052	0.0051	0.0049	0.0048
2.6	0.0047	0.0045	0.0044	0.0043	0.0041	0.004	0.0039	0.0038	0.0037	0.0036
2.7	0.0035	0.0034	0.0033	0.0032	0.0031	0.003	0.0029	0.0028	0.0027	0.0026
2.8	0.0026	0.0025	0.0024	0.0023	0.0023	0.0022	0.0021	0.0021	0.002	0.0019
2.9	0.0019	0.0018	0.0018	0.0017	0.0016	0.0016	0.0015	0.0015	0.0014	0.0014
3.0	0.0013	0.0013	0.0013	0.0012	0.0012	0.0011	0.0011	0.011	0.001	0.001
3.1	0.001	0.0009	0.0009	0.0009	0.0008	0.0008	0.0008	0.0008	0.0007	0.0007
3.2	0.0007	0.0007	0.0006	0.0006	0.0006	0.0006	0.0006	0.0005	0.0005	0.0005
3.3	0.0005	0.0005	0.0005	0.0004	0.0004	0.0004	0.0004	0.0004	0.0004	0.0003
3.4	0.0003	0.0003	0.0003	0.0003	0.0003	0.0003	0.0003	0.0003	0.0003	0.0002

Practise calculating z scores. To be pragmatic we will use a data set of ten numbers, but you need to remember that to use z scores with confidence the data set should be greater than thirty.

A nurse mentor decides she wants to compare the number of times students have given an injection during an A&E ward placement. The values are given in Table 11.2.

TABLE 11.2   Number of injections delivered by a group of student nurses on an A&E ward

Student Nurse	1	2	3	4	5	6	7	8	9	10
Number of Injections	9	3	19	5	7	8	23	5	3	8

What the nurse mentor wants to know is the probability of a student nurse managing to have four opportunities or fewer to deliver an injection (four is a bare minimum that the mentor wants a student to achieve). So, what would you need to know? Look at the equation on p.103. To calculate z for a particular case (value) you need to enter three things (parameters) into the equation. Using the equation to calculate z

$$z = \frac{x - \bar{x}}{S}$$

we have done the calculation below.

Do the top part of the equation first and then divide by the bottom.

$$Z = \frac{4 - 9}{6.72} = -0.75$$

When calculating z scores the minus values tell us if the case is greater or less than the mean. −ve it's less than, +ve it's greater than.

Having calculated the z score (−0.75) for the value 4, you need to look that value up on Table 11.1. This will tell you the proportion of the normal curve that is cut off at this z score. Ignore the sign. How do you look up this value? Go down the first column until you reach 0.7, then go across until you reach 0.05. (If you add 0.7 and 0.05 together you will get 0.75.) Read the value off the table.

With this mean and this SD, the proportion of the population cut off or remaining will be 0.2266 or 23 per cent. So, we are predicting that the proportion of student nurses that achieve four injections or less will be 23 per cent. Clearly this chance is too high and the nurse mentor needs to rethink how this aspect of learning opportunity of the A&E placement needs to be managed.

Clearly, with a sample of ten, it is relatively easy to see what the data are suggesting, but say we had fifty students or even 750 to manage.

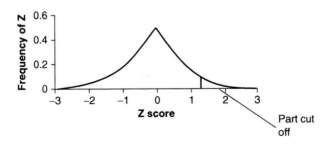

FIGURE 11.2 Normal distribution showing the proportion of the curve cut off at a z score of 1.3

Note two things here about using z scores:

1. To make a prediction about a case in a distribution you only need to know the standard deviation (SD) and the mean.
2. In the example above, see how close our prediction of 23 per cent is to the value that you would have guessed at (probably 20 per cent). These ten numbers are not normally distributed (we just used them for an example). Nevertheless, despite this, the prediction is quite close to reality. This demonstrates an important feature of tests based on the normal distribution, i.e. they tend to be what statisticians call **robust**. That is, you can break some of the assumptions and they will still work.

If you practise the exercise at the end of the book it will help you understand.

Another useful aspect to z scores is that they can be used in reverse, that is say we had a set of data and we wanted to predict the value of a case that would occur at a certain probability or risk level. We will use an example to illustrate this.

Staff nurse Andrew Peters has responsibility for maintaining clean utility supplies within a busy A&E department. He has been informed that the unit has to move to a new building. Inevitably, as with most new buildings, there is less space for storage and Andrew is concerned about the number of sterile dressings that he should be able to stock. Fluctuating demands are placed on A&E departments and so it is difficult to predict just how many sterile dressings may be required during any particular week. Obviously, Andrew could keep a vast stock of dressings but he would have little room for anything else, so clearly he needs to make a risk assessment. The cost of over-stocking is wasted space, while the cost of under-stocking may affect the ability of the department to provide appropriate care for patients. Fortunately, Andrew has collected information on the number of dressings used per week over the last year. His sample size is thus fifty-two, and he has calculated that the mean number of dressings used per week is fifty-eight with an SD of nine. The theoretical normal distribution for this SD and mean is shown below. Now let's say that Andrew wants to be prepared for all but the most extreme circumstances, and he decides he wants to be prepared for 99 per cent of all demand levels. He would then look in the z table for the value of 1 per cent or 0.01. Remember the z table tells us what's left. He must look in the table not at the z scores down the sides.

The z score is about 2.29. Now you need to do some maths. We want to know what case this z score gives us, i.e. how many dressings.

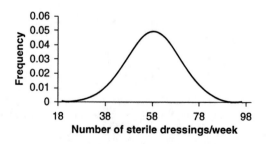

FIGURE 11.3 Theoretical normal distribution for a mean of 58 and standard deviation of 9

To do this we need to put the values we know into the equation we used to calculate z. Remember that s is the symbol given to the standard deviation.

$$z = \frac{x - \overline{x}}{s}$$

In Andrew's example $2.29 = \dfrac{x - 58}{9}$

Andrew must solve the equation for the case value x. To do this multiply both sides of the equation by 9, this gives you 20.61 = x –58, because you can cancel the 9s on the right-hand side of the equation. Then simply take the –58 to the other side of the equation, where it will become a +58, thus we have:

78.61 = x

Thus if Andrew wants a 95 per cent chance of never running out of sterile dressing he needs to keep about seventy-nine in stock.

Having read this chapter and completed the exercises, you should be familiar with the follow ideas and concepts.

- that statistics can be made to make predictions;
- that the SE and confidence intervals are predictions;
- how to calculate SEs and confidence intervals of sample means;
- what the term robust means;

- how to calculate z scores;
- how to use z scores to make predictions;
- that the SE and confidence intervals predict how close a sample mean is to a population mean;
- be aware of the central limit theorem.

---

1. In the Symphadiol experiment the mean of the heights in the control group is 179 cm. Calculate the standard deviation, the SE and the 95 per cent confidence limits of the mean.
2. For each of the calculations in question 1 describe what each statistic is telling you.
3. Bernard Smith is a community nurse working with a needle exchange programme. There is concern that the mobile unit occasionally runs out of clean needles. Bernard has recorded how many clean needles are used each night; he has calculated the mean to be seventy-six and the SD to be twenty. (a) What healthcare problems do you think running out of needles might create? (b) How might running out of needles undermine the programme? (c) Calculate how many needles Bernard needs to stock in order to be (i) 95 per cent and (ii) 65 per cent certain of not running out of needles.

EXERCISES

12

Testing for differences between means

Areas of learning covered in this chapter

- How do I test to see if there is a difference between means?
- What are the F, z and t tests?
- When should F, z and t tests be used?
- What is the difference between a one- and two-tailed test?

We have seen how we can use statistics to make predictions. Now we are going to see how we can use them to predict if the differences between two sets of results could have occurred by chance.

Let's say that you have set up your study, you have a control and an experimental group, and the experimental group is subject to an intervention. You have been measuring patients' post-operative recovery rates on surgical wards in relation to having a new therapy. In this therapy patients are played tapes of their favourite music whilst undergoing surgery. In this study the variable being measured is the time taken to recover; thus our dependent variable is time. The independent variable will be the treatment group. Patients could have been ascribed to either the study group or the control group.

Box 12.1 Good design

What steps would you take to ensure that your control group was representative?

Having collected your data the first thing you should do is plot the data. This will allow you to get a handle on what your data feels like. You may want to plot the data as frequency histograms

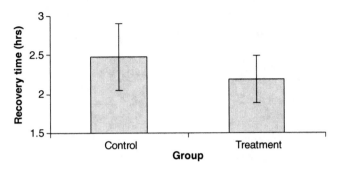

FIGURE 12.1   Mean post-operative recovery time of two groups of patients. The treatment group were played tapes of their favourite music

and also as bar charts, with bars showing the variation. Bars normally show either the range, the SE or the SD. Sometimes, more than one statistic is shown (see Chapter 7).

You've now plotted the data. You notice that the treatment group has a faster recovery time. You will also notice by plotting a histogram if there are any unusual results (outliers).

So, there is a difference between the mean recovery time of the two groups. The question we need to ask is how likely is it that this difference has occurred by chance, i.e. is it likely that the difference is simply due to sampling errors (Chapter 9). Remember the data you used in Box 11.2. These data were all drawn from the same population but the differences between the means were all different. The difference was due to sampling error. The question we are asking when we are testing to see if the observed result is probably due to chance is: do these means come from the same population (in which case there would be no difference between the population means) or do they come from two separate populations (the difference between the populations being the impact of the treatment)?

> ## Box 12.2   When do you need a test?
>
> Based on the descriptives, when might you decide not to do a statistical test?

12.1 The *F* test

There are a whole group of tests associated with this problem. In this chapter we will look at statistics called *F*, student's *t* and *z*. The *t* test is probably one of the most often used tests. Like most tests they have rules about when they should and should not be used. In fact, the art of applying statistics is to know when to use a particular test, i.e. which rules apply to which. You could liken this to some therapies. For example, as practitioners you may not understand fully how a particular drug works, but based on a set of symptoms you know when to apply it and when not to. So it is with statistics. We need to know which to apply and when, and even if we don't follow the maths we can select the correct test from a computer package.

Box 12.3 Exploring the tests

Look through a few quantitative research papers that you have access to. Which statistics are used most often?

The rules for the tests F, z and t are the following:

- the dependent variable must be measured on the interval scale;
- the samples must come from a normally distributed population;
- with respect to z and t, the **variance** of the samples must be equal.[1]

We will look at the variance first, as this is the basis of the F test. The variance is just another measure of variation; in fact, it is simply the SD squared (s^2). It is used in a large number of statistical tests.

The F test or, to give its full name, the **F test for equality of variance** tests to find if the variances of the two samples are equal or, as we should say, 'not significantly different'. Why is this important? If the variances are different, it tells us that the shapes of the normal distributions that the populations are drawn upon differ markedly. If the shapes are very different then it is unlikely that the mean of one sample is drawn from the same sample as the other. The shape of the distributions is as important as the means.

As you can see from Figure 12.2, the shapes of these two distributions look different. If the shapes are actually statistically different then there is little point in testing to see if the means come from the same population because quite clearly they do not. Thus, it is good practice to apply an F test first before testing to see if there is a significant difference between the means.

The F test statistic is calculated as:

$$F = \frac{\text{greater variance}}{\text{lesser variance}}$$

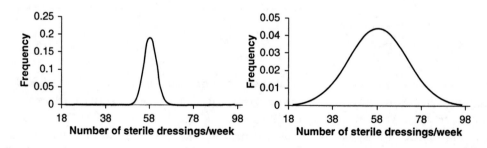

FIGURE 12.2   Clearly the distributions of these two samples are very different

---

[1] As you become more knowledgeable you will find there are ways around this problem

The symbol for the variance is s^2

If the shape of the two distributions of the samples is identical, then F will equal one. The greater the difference between them the larger F will be. But how do we know when to say that F is so big that the difference between them is **significant**? This comes back to the idea of probability. First, we need to decide what level of probability we are working at. We said previously (in Chapter 10) that it's normal to work at P = 0.05, i.e. if the chance of getting a certain value of F is as extreme as 5 per cent (one in twenty) we say the result is significant. With this, F test (known as the F test for equality of variance) we work at the 0.01 level (1 per cent or one in 100).

If the chance of the particular value of F is greater than 0.01 we say that the two distributions are *not* significantly different and we should carry on to do either the z test or the **student's t test**. If the chance is *less* than 0.01, we say they are significantly different. The chance of obtaining a particular value of F will depend on the sizes of the samples.

For example, mental health nurse Ungamba Maliba is conducting some research into the impact of the drug Mindrenew (a fictitious name) on the recall speed of patients with mild Alzheimer's disease. He measures the mean ($\bar{x}$) response of the control group as 180 seconds and the SD as thirty-two seconds. The mean of the treatment group is 180 seconds and the SD sixty-three. Thirty-two participants took part in each group.

Box 12.4

Record the forearm length of a group of males and a group of females.

- For each group, compute the mean, SD and variance.
- Compute the F statistic for equality of variance.
- State the null and alternative hypothesis.

Is there an effect of the treatment? Do the samples eminate from different populations? First, you would do the F test:

$$F = \frac{\text{greater variance}}{\text{lesser variance}} = \frac{3969}{1024} \qquad F = 3.87$$

Having found the value of F you must now compare it to the value in the F table, at the 0.01 level of probability (see Appendix 3). Looking at this table notice that the top row is labelled v_1 and that first column is labelled v_2. These refer to the sample size of each of the two samples −1. In other words:

$$v_1 = 32 - 1 = 31$$
$$v_2 = 32 - 1 = 31$$

Now find the column in the table that starts with a value close to 31 and the row where the value is also close to 31. Note the value where these columns and rows cross each other. The value you should find is about 2.36. Because our calculated value is greater than this value we can say that the there is a **statistically significant difference** in the shape of the two distributions and therefore they are likely to be samples from two different populations.

> If you use a statistical computer package, for most tests the computer will look up the value and compare it with the test statistic for you.

> What could Ungamba Maliba conclude about the impact of Mindrenew on Alzheimer's disease?

Note a good rule of thumb here. When we compare the value given by a statistical test to that in a table, in general if the calculated value is *larger* than the value in the table then the result is significant.

If we find that the result is not statistically different, we say there is *no significant difference*. This means that whilst the actual recorded values may be different there is a high probability that this difference has occurred by chance.

12.2 Testing for difference between the means (z and t test)

z test

Let's say that in a study the *F* test came up with the answer that there was no statistically significant difference between the two samples.

The z test is not a test you will see quoted very often, as most researchers incorrectly opt for the *t* test. This is partly because most computer packages do not carry a facility for doing the z test and also any error is unlikely to affect the conclusion of the test. The z test should be used if your sample sizes are large, and when you are comparing the means of two samples.

If the null hypothesis (no difference) is correct then as we said before any difference between the mean is simply due to sampling error. But how big does the difference need to be before we say that they are significantly different?

To answer this question we turn to z scores again. If the difference is greater than a z of 1.96 then it is significantly different at the 5 per cent level (2.58 at the 1 per cent level).

But which z, as both distributions may have different SDs? The answer is the z here refers to the *standard error of the difference between the two means*.

To use statistics you do not need to know how the test works, just which one to use when; but understanding a procedure will help your development as a practitioner. We include the next section just to show how the test works.

Look back at the data shown in Figure 12.1. Let's say they are from the same population, i.e. the treatment had no effect, then there should ideally be no difference between the mean, but we know that because of error this ideal is unlikely.

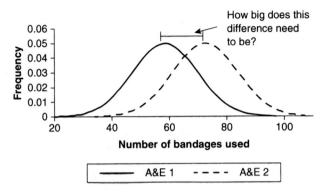

FIGURE 12.3 Two distributions are shown of data on the number of bandages used on two A&E departments. Clearly there is a difference in the number used, but is this difference statistically significant?

Imagine that you drew two more samples from the population. There would again be a difference. We record this difference and then repeat again and again. We would generate a sample of differences, differences between samples. If we plot this sample of differences as a frequency histogram we would find perhaps to our surprise that it was normally distributed, with a mean population of 0. Of course like other normal distributions, this distribution of differences has a standard deviation; this standard deviation is called the standard error of the difference.

The z test statistic asks: is the difference between the two sample means greater than the standard error of the difference? And, if so, how big? The statistic z is calculated as the difference between the sample means minus the population mean. (The population mean of this sample of differences will always be 0 if the two samples are in reality drawn from the same population.)

Box 12.5

1. Using your data collected for the exercise in Box 12.4, perform a z test.
2. What is the null hypothesis? What is the alternative hypothesis?
3. What do you conclude?

The difference in the means is then divided by the standard error of the difference. In this case, the mathematical formula does look simper than the words:

$$z = \frac{\left(\bar{x}_1 - \bar{x}_2\right) - 0}{\text{SE of the difference}}$$

(Equation 1)

where $\bar{x}_1$ = the mean of sample 1

and

where $\bar{x}_2$ = the mean of sample 2

It doesn't matter which sample you decide to be sample 1 and which sample 2.

What we haven't told you yet is how to find the SE of the difference. Obviously, as you have only two samples to work with it would be difficult to produce a frequency distribution. So, we have to estimate the value based on the variance of the two samples. The formula to calculate the SE of the difference is given below:

$$SE \ of \ diff. = \sqrt{\frac{s_1^2}{n_1} + \frac{s_2^2}{n_2}}$$

where s is the standard deviation.

Given that you can now calculate the SE of the difference you can use equation 1 to calculate z. If a value you calculate is greater than 1.96 you can say that the means are significantly different at the $P < 0.05$ (5 per cent) level. If the value is greater than 2.58 you can say that the means are significantly different at the $P < 0.01$ (1 per cent) level (< is the symbol for less than). Here, we have introduced the idea of different levels of significance. The levels we normally talk of are $P < 0.05$, $P < 0.01$, $P < 0.001$ and $P < 0.0001$. The lower the level of P the greater confidence you have in your result not having occurred by chance. These levels are arbitrary and it is becoming common with the advent of computers, to quote the exact **P value** given by the computer package.

When we say there is a significant difference, we are *rejecting* the null hypothesis. This is because the chance of getting a result (a z value) as high as this is very low.

Box 12.6   Reminder

Remember, your first steps would be to plot out your raw data, and check that they were normally distributed. You would then plot the means on a bar chart, showing the extent of the variation using error bars. Then you would perform an F test. If the F test indicates that the sample sizes are not significantly different then you should proceed with a test that looks at the means. As the sample size is large here, we opt for the z test.

An example

An occupational health department has decided to investigate if a new shift pattern results in more or fewer incidents of back injury. They have decided to use a controlled study and half the workforce operate the old shift pattern (control group) whilst the other half operate the new system (experimental or treatment group). They measure the reported back pain per week in the two groups. The dependent variable is thus change in reported back pain per week. The independent variable is the experimental groups (control and treatment). The results are shown in Table 12.1

TABLE 12.1 Mean results and descriptive statistics from a study on the impact of shift pattern on back injuries

| Sample | No. of reports of back pain | | Sample size (n) |
	Mean ($\bar{x}$)	Standard deviation(s)	
Control	21	6	182
Treatment	18	5	196

Step 1: calculate the standard error of the difference:

$$SE \text{ of } diff. = \sqrt{\frac{s_1^2}{n_1} + \frac{s_2^2}{n_2}} = \sqrt{\frac{6_1^2}{182_1} + \frac{5_2^2}{196_2}} = \sqrt{\frac{36}{182_1} + \frac{25}{196_2}}$$

$$= \sqrt{\frac{61}{378}} = \sqrt{0.16} = 0.40$$

Step 2: calculate the difference between the means:

$$= \left(\bar{x}_1 - \bar{x}_2\right) - 0 = (21 - 18) - 0 = 3$$

Step 3: calculate z, i.e. divide the result from step 2 by that from step 1:

$$z = \frac{3}{0.40} = 7.5$$

As z is bigger than both 1.96 and 2.54 we can reject the null hypothesis (no difference) and say that the means *are* significantly different and conclude that the introduction of the new shift pattern reduces the reported incidence of back pain.

Note that, having come to the statistical conclusion, i.e. is the difference significant or not, we can then move to the conclusion of the study, i.e. was the treatment effective.

The student's t test

This test tends to appear in all introductory tests on statistics and is still probably one of the most used tests. It is particularly of use for small-scale studies where the questions being asked are simple and the sample size low.

> The person who invents a test often names them. The person who invented the student's t test was prevented by his employer from giving it his own name so he called it the 'student's'.

With small samples it becomes difficult to make a reliable judgement or test on whether or not the samples are normally distributed. The t test makes the assumption that the parent population from which the samples are drawn are normally distributed. It also assumes that variances of the two samples are similar and that the data are measured on the interval scale.

The t test assumes that the samples themselves are not distributed normally but distributed according the t distribution. This distribution is like a flattened normal distribution with long tails. It uses a new statistic called the pooled variance. The pooled variance is used to calculate the SE of the difference as used in the z test. We won't go in to the theory here but we will show you how the t test is carried out.

> Most computer packages do not have a facility to conduct a z test. Use a t test instead – the result will be equivalent.

The pooled variance is calculated as:

$$S_c^2 = \frac{n_1 s_1^2 + n_2 s_2^2}{n_1 + n_2 - 2}$$

Here S_c^2 is the pooled variance

n_1 is the sample size for sample 1

n_2 is the sample size for sample 2

s_1^2 is the variance for sample 1

s_2^2 is the variance for sample 2

t itself is given by the equation:

$$t = \frac{(\bar{x}_1 - \bar{x}_2) - 0}{S_c \times \sqrt{\frac{1}{n_1} + \frac{1}{n_2}}}$$

Here S_c is the square root of S_c^2. The rest of the symbols you have met before.

Box 12.7

1. Using your data collected for the exercise in Box 12.2, perform a t test.
2. What is the null hypothesis? What is the alternative hypothesis?
3. What do you conclude?
4. Is a z test or a t test more appropriate?

An example

Mary Smith is a physiotherapist who is working as part of a multi-professional health care team treating osteoarthritis. She is interested in evaluating the effect of a new manipulation therapy regime on the recovery of patients who have had surgery to insert artificial knee joints.

She has obtained consent from the ethics committee to conduct her research and sixty patients have volunteered. Unfortunately just twenty-eight of these patients are within the exact **target group** that the team is interested in (for example correct age and sex). Fourteen patients are allocated to the treatment group and fourteen to the control group.

As a measure of recovery, Mary has chosen to use the angle of contraction that patients are able to achieve when moving from a standing to a crouching position without pain. The dependent variable is thus the angle. The independent variable is the experimental group, either control or treatment.

TABLE 12.2 Mean results and descriptive statistics from a study on the impact of a new manipulation on recovery from knee surgery

	Angle of contraction		Sample Size
Sample	Mean ($\bar{x}$)	Standard Deviation(s)	(n)
Control	11.2	3.12	14
Treatment	10.3	2.54	14

Example from the literature 12.1   Using a t test

The t test is a relatively common statistical test. In their paper that examines whether or not intensity of therapy influences an individual's recovery from stroke, Sivenius et al. (1985) use a t test to determine the significance of the difference between the means of their two independent groups of stroke (cranial vascular accident) victims. One group received intensive therapy, whilst the other the 'normal' therapy.

They compared the efficacy of the two groups using a variable based on scores of the participant's motor function and activities of daily living (ADL). These scores were compared using t tests. The authors also use a test called an analysis of covariance (ANCOVA) – this test is quite complex and is not covered by this book.

As you read this article and compare it to the approach suggested in this book you may notice a few discrepancies. The authors for example do not conduct a preliminary F test to look for equality of variance. This is probably because the sample sizes in the two groups are very similar. Nevertheless, this a check worth doing which is omitted.

The authors also do not seem to have checked to make sure that their data do not have a distribution that significantly deviates from the normal distribution. This is a particularly important check to do when working with data composed of subjective scores rather than direct measurements. As the level of statistical significant difference between the two treatment groups is relatively low we would do this check. This failure to examine the distribution of the data would lead us to treat Sivenius et al. (1985) with caution.

(Continued)

(Continued)

Finally, given the sample size (approximately fifty in each group) the choice of test looks slightly odd. Why not do a z test instead? In fact, however, many computer packages do not provide an easy facility to compute a z test and with larger samples the t test will give the same result as the z test.

Sivenius et al.'s (1985) paper is freely available at http://stroke.ahajournals.org/content/16/6/928.full.pdf. It is a relatively old paper, but we have used this work to illustrate the use of the t test in a real study, not as an example of current health practice.

As with the z test, having collected the data the first steps would be to plot the data, then to conduct an F test. If the F test indicates that the variance is similar (not significantly different) then you would proceed with the t test. We use a t test here because the sample size is small, but we have a good idea that the parent population would be normally distributed.

S^2 (the variance) is the standard deviation squared.

Step 1: calculate the pooled variance.

$$S_c^2 = \frac{n_1 s_1^2 + n_2 s_2^2}{n_1 + n_2 - 2}$$

$$= \frac{14 \times 3.12^2 + 14 \times 2.54^2}{14 + 14 - 2} = \frac{14 \times 9.73 + 14 \times 6.45}{26}$$

$$= \frac{136.22 + 90.3}{26} = \frac{136.22 + 90.3}{26} = \frac{226.55}{26} = 8.71$$

Step 2: calculate t.

$$t = \frac{(\bar{x}_1 - \bar{x}_2) - 0}{S_c \times \sqrt{\dfrac{1}{n_1} + \dfrac{1}{n_2}}} =$$

$$\frac{11.2 - 10.3}{9.71 \times \sqrt{\dfrac{1}{14} + \dfrac{1}{14}}} = \frac{0.9}{9.71 \times \sqrt{0.071 + 0.071}} = \frac{0.9}{9.71 \times 0.142}$$

$$= \frac{0.9}{1.382} = 0.65$$

So $t = 0.65$. You now need to look up this value in the t distribution table using the sample size of 28. However, when using a t test and many other tests, rather than using the actual sample size we use something called the **degrees of freedom**. In the case of the student's t test the degrees of freedom are the total sample size −2 (because there are two experimental groups). So, we have 28 − 2 degrees of freedom or 26. If you go to Table 3 in Appendix 3, you will see degrees of freedom, or d.f., down the first column and significance levels across the top.

Mary Smith is conducting a clinical study and therefore feels it is appropriate to work at the 0.01 (1 per cent) level. Look down the 0.01 column until it meets the row for 26 degrees of freedom. The value is 2.779. Our calculated value is much smaller than this

As our value is smaller than that in the table, we can say that there is no statistically significant difference. Mary Smith can therefore conclude that the new therapy regime does not result in a significant improvement in the recovery of her patients with respect to the measured variable at the time of testing.

Box 12.8 Expressing the results

When you describe the result of a statistical test you must tell the reader the type of test used, the value of the test statistic, the sample size and at what probability level the result was significant (or not). In Mary Smith's study, we would say there was no statistically significant difference between the control and the treatment group (Student's: $t = 2.78$ n = 28 $P > 0.01$).

When looking at the detail of the t test you will see that although the maths is not that complex it involves a number of calculations. You will also realize that performing all these calculations by hand is laborious and prone to error, hence the evolution of the statistical computer package. We would recommend that you use a computer package whenever they are available.

12.3 Power

We have said that the t test is designed for small sample sizes, but how small? You can perform the calculations on very small samples, but in practice as your sample size becomes smaller your tests will tend to get the outcome of 'no significant difference' more often even if your treatment in reality has an effect. This is because as your sample size becomes smaller the **power** of the statistical test becomes less. Power in statistical terms means the ability to show a statistically significant result if there is indeed one.

Contrast the term *power* with that of *robust.*

12.4 Paired *t* test

Another type of *t* test you will come across is called the paired *t* test. This test is a member of a type of test known as the **repeat measures designs**. The tests we have described so far all involve situations were we have allocated participants to one group or another (control or treatment). What if we want to see the impact of a treatment before and then after an intervention? This would be an example of a repeat measures design because we would repeat the measurements on the same participants.

When we do this type of study, we actually have less error to contend with because using the same participants removes all the error associated with using two different groups of people, i.e. we no longer need to take into account the natural variation in response that occurs between the participants, and we can focus on the difference before and after. The maths of the test is slightly different but the principle is identical. Again the variables must be measured using the interval or ratio scale.

Example

Mohammed Dhauba, a consultant nurse in a cardiac outpatients unit, is concerned that most of his patients' diastolic blood pressure is higher on initial measurements than on subsequent measurements. This difference could be for several reasons. He decides to investigate whether or not it is true and to determine the significance of his findings for his patients.

He measures the blood pressure of twenty patients within ten minutes of them entering the outpatients department and then *repeats* the measurement two hours later. Because he repeats the measurement on the same participants, he knows he needs to use a repeat measures design test. Because he has two experimental groups (after ten minutes and then two hours later) and his sample is rather small he selects a paired *t* test. Here the **dependent variable** is blood pressure and the **independent variable** is time. The summary statistics are shown in Table 12.3.

The mechanics of the paired t test retreats back to using the SE of the difference as in the *z* test. Obviously if you are measuring the same person, if there is no effect of the time interval then the difference between the measurements will be 0. Thus, the mean of all the participants' differences will be 0 if there is no effect. However, because of error we know it's unlikely that even if the treatment has no effect the means will equal 0, but how big does that deviation need to be? This is exactly the same question that we posed with respect to the *z* test and the answer is the same, the only difference being that this time we can actually calculate the mean of the differences and calculate the SE of these differences.

TABLE 12.3 Mean results and descriptive statistics from a study on the difference between initial and subsequent measures of diastolic blood pressure

Sample	Mean ($\bar{x}$) diastolic BP (mmHg)	Standard deviation(s)	Sample size (n)
10 mins	94.23	10.17	20
2 hours	85.58	8.19	20

In the paired t test, it is the differences that need to be normally distributed not the measurement variables themselves.

The formula for the paired t test is as below:

$$t = \frac{\Sigma d}{\sqrt{\dfrac{n\Sigma d^2 - (\Sigma d)^2}{n-1}}}$$

Again, the formula looks complex, but taken step by step it really is not that bad.

Here d refers to the difference between the initial measurement for an individual and the subsequent one. The symbol Σ (an upper-case sigma) means the sum of; you met it in the chapter on descriptive statistics (Chapter 6). Σd means all the differences between the two measurements of the individuals added together. To do this test by hand you need all the raw data.

TABLE 12.4 The differences between initial measures of diastolic blood pressure and those taken two hours later

Individual participant	BP after 10 mins mmHZ	BP after 2 hrs mmbarHz	d	d²
1	109	88	+21	441
2	104	84	+20	400
3	84	86	−2	4
4	80	84	−4	16
5	90	75	+15	225
6	107	81	+26	676
7	106	92	+14	196
8	98	86	+12	144
9	78	90	−12	144
10	89	82	+7	49
11	91	77	+14	196
12	85	95	−10	100
13	87	88	−1	1
14	101	84	+17	289
15	94	88	+6	36
16	87	75	+12	144
17	85	94	−9	81
18	111	73	+38	1444
19	103	82	+21	441
20	97	107	−10	100
			$\Sigma d = 175$	$\Sigma d^2 = 5127$

When doing a paired t test there is no need to test for equality of the variance.

Step 1: prepare a table of results and calculate Σd and Σd^2.

Step 2: calculate $(\Sigma d)^2$ in this case 175^2 which equals 30625.

Step 3: feed the values in to the equation.

$$t = \frac{\Sigma d}{\sqrt{\dfrac{n\Sigma d^2 - (\Sigma d)^2}{n-1}}} = \frac{175}{\sqrt{\dfrac{(20 \times 5127) - 30625}{20 - 1}}} = \frac{175}{\sqrt{\dfrac{102540 - 30625}{19}}}$$

$$= \frac{175}{\sqrt{\dfrac{102540 - 30625}{19}}} = \frac{175}{\sqrt{3595.75}} = \frac{175}{59.96} = 2.91$$

Look up your value of t in Appendix 3, Table 3, using the appropriate number of degrees of freedom, in this case nineteen.

The degrees of freedom used in this test equal $n - 1$. The value of n in the paired t test as in all statistical tests is the sample size. You may be thinking, 'But I have made forty measurements'. However, because the test works on the difference between the two measures on the same subject, you actually only have twenty samples of differences.

So, you look up 2.91 in the table for 19 degrees of freedom. 2.91 is greater than the value of 2.093 for the $P = 0.05$ level of significance and also for that of 2.861 for the $P = 0.01$ level. We can thus say that there is a statistical difference in the diastolic BP between the measurement time intervals.

Therefore, we reject the **null hypothesis** that there is no difference between the diastolic BP of patients measured at ten minutes and two hours after arrival at the outpatients clinic. We conclude that a time interval of one hour and fifty minutes between an initial BP measurement on arrival at the clinic and a subsequent measurement leads to a significantly different result being recorded.

Example from the literature 12.2   A paired t test

Paired t tests are often used when taking more than one measure of the same variable from the same individual. Chen et al. (2013) used a paired t test when they compared differing positions (prone and supine) for the radiotherapy of Asian women with breast cancer. They used a t test to help compare the shape of breasts in differing positions. The shape of the breast influences both the effectiveness of the radiotherapy treatment and also the extent to which surrounding organs may be affected. The study concluded that the prone position was better. You can see how the paired t test was used by looking at Table 1 of their research paper, which you can find at: http://jrr.oxfordjournals.org/content/early/2013/03/15/jrr.rrt019.full.pdf.

Bigger or smaller, one or two tails?

One aspect of statistical testing that always tends to add confusion is the problem of tails. You may see written 'We use a two-tailed t test', but what does this mean?

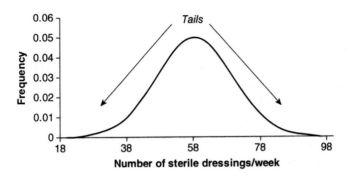

FIGURE 12.4

Let's recall the normal distribution from the study in Chapter 11. As with all normal-like distribution it has two tails. This is where the term **two-tailed test** comes from.

Box 12.9   Recap

Use the z and t tests when you are looking to see if there is a significant difference between the means of two samples.

Use them only where the samples are normally distributed (z test or you suspect that the parent population is normally distributed).

Use them only for variables that are measured on the interval scale.

Check that the variances are equal; use an F test for equality of variance.

Decide whether or not you will opt for a one-tailed or a two-tailed test.

When we do a test we are trying to determine if our result is extreme and so are asking if the test statistic or result lie in the tails of the distribution, if it fits. Does it belong with the distribution of this population or is it so extreme in all probability it belongs with another?

But because the tails are at both ends, it means we are looking for values both much smaller than the mean and much bigger. In this case, in terms of the hypotheses we are simply looking for a difference, i.e. the null hypothesis is that there is no difference. The alternative to the null H_1 is that there is a difference.

But what if we suspect that our treatment (or intervention) will have a big effect in a particular direction, such as decreasing the prevalence of a disease or increasing the recovery rate. Indeed, in many health care studies we are looking for a difference in a particular direction. In this case, we are looking for extreme values in one end of the tail only. To convert from a two-tailed test to a one-tailed test is easy: simply divide the probability level (P) by two.

- If you are just looking for a difference, use a two-tailed test.
- If you think your intervention will increase the measured variable, use a one-tailed test.
- If you think your intervention will decrease the measured variable, use a one-tailed test.

In the example used to explain the paired t test clearly there is prior belief that BPs recorded two hours after arrival will be lower than those recorded soon after arrival. This is a clear example where a **one-tailed test** could be used. When applied to the example the result is significant at a lower level of probability, i.e. 0.01 divided by two, which equals 0.05. Thus, the result has a higher level of significance. In some cases, the decision to use a one- or two-tailed test can affect whether the null hypothesis is accepted or rejected. Therefore, *if in doubt use a two-tailed test.*

Having read this chapter and completed the exercises, you should be familiar with the following ideas and concepts:

- how and when to perform an f test for equality of variance;
- how and when to perform a z and student's t tests;
- how to perform a paired t test;

- the rules that restrict the use of the t test;
- the difference between a one- and two-tailed test;
- when to use a one-tailed test;
- when to use a two-tailed test.

EXERCISES

1. Using the data from the Symphadiol study plot a histogram using the descriptive statistics for weight loss for group 1 (control) and group 2.
2. State the hypothesis and null hypothesis.
3. You are looking to see if the weight loss of the treatment group is greater than that of the control. Perform an appropriate statistical test(s) on this sample.
4. Give your reasons for your choice of test.
5. Clearly state the conclusion of your test.
6. Using the data in Table 12.5 suggest whether or not biology lectures had a significant impact on the performance of Year 1 nursing studies undergraduates in a biology examination. (a) What explanations could account for this result? (b) Do you think the lectures were of benefit, should the students attend? (c) Did you use a one- or two-tailed test, and why?

TABLE 12.5

Individual	Exam Result Before Lectures	Exam Result After Lectures
1	34.5	37.5
2	37.2	40.2
3	43.0	42.0
4	48.8	51.8
5	49.6	52.6
6	50.8	50.8
7	51.2	54.2
8	51.5	54.5
9	52.5	55.5
10	63.4	62.4
11	64.6	67.6

13

Errors and ANOVAs

Areas of learning covered in this chapter

- What are type I and type II errors?
- What can be done to reduce Type 1 errors?
- How are ANOVAs performed?
- When do I use a repeat measures design?

In the previous chapter we looked at tests based on the normal distribution designed to see if there is a difference between two treatment groups, but what if you have more than two groups? Say you have a control group at two different levels of a treatment. In this case you can't use a *t* test and must use a type of test that belongs to a group called **ANOVA**, which is shorthand for *analysis of variance*. There are several types of ANOVA but they have evolved to deal with a certain type of statistical error.

Statistical errors

If we choose the wrong type of statistical test we are likely to commit either a type I or a type II error.

A **type I error** occurs when you reject the null hypothesis when it should have been accepted.

A **type II error** is when we reject the alternative hypothesis when it should have been accepted.

Type I and type II errors are opposites. As you reduce the likelihood of a type I error the chance of a type II error increases. In general, we tend to select test that will *reduce* the chance of a type I error, so a cautious approach is adopted. For example, we have said previously that in many medical studies the significance level is set at $P = 0.01$.

Do not spend too much energy trying to remember which is which, just work on understanding what they mean. You can look up which is which when you need to.

t tests, errors and ANOVAs

We have said that you need an ANOVA when you have more than two groups. Let's look at why.

Imagine we are doing a study where we have a control group (C) and two treatment groups (TI and TII). We want to see if their means are significantly different. If we use a *t* test then we need to do several tests. We must test:

C against TI;

TI against TII;

TII against C.

Perhaps this is not too much trouble if using a computer or even a calculator but if you had five treatment groups you would need to do ten tests. Even if you are prepared to stand the boredom, and manage not to make any calculation errors, you will commit a statistical error.

Box 13.1   Errors

If you set your accepted value at 0.01 (1 per cent) then you would have a one in 100 chance of getting it wrong. So a simple solution looks to be to increase the significance level. Unfortunately as type I and type II errors are opposites, as we decrease the chance of making a type I error the chance of producing a type II error increases.

This is because if you set your significance level at the normally accepted value of $P = 0.05$ (5 per cent), once every twentieth test (on average) you will get it wrong and commit a type I error. But if, as in the case above, where we have five treatment groups you perform ten *t* tests the chance of one of these being wrong goes up to one in two (i.e. 0.05×10). So we need a way around this problem. The solution is to use an ANOVA.

Box 13.2   Robust and powerful

1. ANOVA is described as both a *powerful* and *robust technique*. What do these terms mean?

What ANOVA does is allow us to compare the means of several treatment groups at the same time without having to worry about adjusting *P* values or increasing the chance of type II errors. It does this because it compares all the treatment groups in a single test. As you can imagine, the number of calculations needed to perform an ANOVA is quite large. However, with the advent of computers the use of ANOVA has become much more common and many more ANOVA-type tests have been designed. In this chapter we will look at two types of ANOVA.

The ANOVA

We will first describe the theory behind the ANOVA and then give one example, which we will work through. We will include the mathematical computation so that you can get an idea of how it works. In general it is better to use a computer as they make fewer errors than humans. We suggest that you focus on the structure of the tests and interpreting the output. The type of ANOVA that we will describe is called the one-way analysis of variance.

Box 13.3 Statistics computer packages

SPSS, MINITAB and MSExcel can all help you to analyse data using the one-way ANOVA described here.

Criteria to be met before doing an ANOVA test:

1. The data of each treatment group are derived from a normal distribution.
2. The data were measured on an interval scale.
3. The variance between each group is not significantly different (there are ways around this one).
4. The sample groups are measured **independently** of each other (see below).

Box 13.4 What is meant by

- normal distribution?
- interval scale?
- variance?

How it works

First, here are some data. The data set is smaller than would be normally used for ANOVA but we will use it to help us examine the ANOVA. The data in Table 13.1 are from a study to examine whether the pre-natal fitness level of primip women significantly affects the duration of

TABLE 13.1 Duration of labour in primip women aged 28–32 at three different levels of fitness (level 1 = low, level 2 = medium, level 3 = high)

Fitness level 1	Fitness level 2	Fitness level 3
20	34	16
32	12	15
14	23	22
15	10	10

labour. A primip is a term given to a woman who is in her first pregnancy. We want to compare the means of these three groups, but we can't use a *t* test. So we must opt for an ANOVA.

> ANOVA seeks to determine how much of the variation in data sets can be attributed to error and how much can be attributed to the factor or treatment under study.

The ANOVA test looks at the source of variation in the overall data set and tries to apportion it to different aspects of the data. Once the variation has been allocated it is then possible to see if the differences between the sample groups are significant. The sources of variation in the data are the variability that occurs *within* a sample group and the variability that occurs *between* the groups.

TABLE 13.2 Variation within and between groups

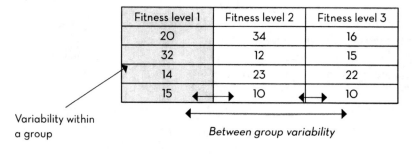

Variability within a group

Between group variability

We can say that:

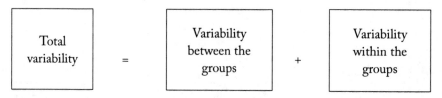

We are interested in the between group variation, i.e. that which has occurred because of the fitness level. The rest of the variation, i.e. that within the groups, we regard as error. The variability between groups will reflect the error that occurs within the groups and any additional variability caused by the treatment (in this case fitness level).

If there is no difference between the groups, i.e. the null hypothesis is correct, then we would expect there to be just as much variation between the groups as there is within the groups. If the between-group variation is more than the within-group variation then we know that the treatment has had an effect; and this is the simple logic behind the ANOVA test.

Box 13.5

1. What are the causes of the within-group variation, i.e. why do the cases of samples show variation?
2. What are the causes of the between-group variation?
3. What is F is a measure of?

The test statistic produced by the ANOVA is F, a statistic we have seen before, and the measure of variation we use is the variance. Hence the name of the test, the analysis of variance.

If we compute the within-group variance and compare it to the between-group variance then F will equal 1 if the null hypothesis is correct. If F is significantly different from 1 we know that the means are significantly different, and the level of fitness (treatment groups) had an effect.

Box 13.6 When to use a one-way ANOVA

- You are comparing the difference between more than two sample groups.
- The data in each of your groups is normally distributed.
- Your data are measured on an interval scale.
- Each case is measured independently.

The procedure for calculating the ANOVA by hand is longwinded; unless you do not have access to a computer, I would not recommend it. It is probably worth doing by hand once or twice as this will help you grasp how the procedure works and how ANOVAs are presented.

An example

In this example, Martha Jones, a physiotherapist, is interested in the impact of the use of a new walking frame on her patients with impaired hip mobility. She has decided to test the new frame at two levels of exercise and use her old frame with the normal level of exercise as a control. Martha uses the distance the patient can walk unassisted as a measure of the effectiveness of the treatments (Table 13.3).

TABLE 13.3 Distance walked by patients (meters) with impaired hip mobility, following various treatment regimes

Old Frame		New Frame Exercise Level 1	New Frame Exercise Level 2
	16.1	22.3	13.2
	17.7	20.5	20.8
	20.6	21.3	22.2
	10.4	26.7	16.3
	20.3	16.3	13.7
	14.9	29.0	11.9
	11.5	24.4	14.1
	14.7	23.7	10.6
	15.3	23.5	15.8
	17.4	19.5	15.9
Mean	15.89	22.72	15.46
Standard Deviation	3.32	3.63	3.67

TABLE 13.4 Statistical summary of the data from Table 13.3

Group 1 (GP1) Old Frame	Group 2 (GP2) New Frame Exercise Level 1	Group 3 (GP3) New Frame Exercise Level 2	Totals
12.1	22.3	13.2	
15.7	20.5	20.8	
18.6	21.3	22.2	
9.4	26.7	16.3	
18.3	16.3	13.7	
12.9	29.0	11.9	
9.5	24.4	14.1	
12.7	23.7	10.6	
13.3	23.5	15.8	
15.4	19.5	15.9	
$n = 10$	$n = 10$	$n = 10$	$n_{tot} = 30$
$\bar{X} = 13.79$	$\bar{X} = 22.72$	$\bar{X} = 15.46$	
$s = 3.21$	$s = 3.63$	$s = 3.67$	
$S^2 = 10.27$	$S^2 = 13.15$	$S^2 = 13.45$	
$\Sigma x = 137.9$	$\Sigma x = 227.2$	$\Sigma x = 154.6$	$\Sigma x_{tot} = 519.70$
$(\Sigma x)^2 = 19016.4$	$(\Sigma x)^2 = 51619.8$	$(\Sigma x)^2 = 23890.8$	
$\Sigma x^2 = 1994.11$	$\Sigma x^2 = 5280.36$	$\Sigma x^2 = 2762.4$	$\Sigma x^2_{tot} = 10036.9$

Again, we will assume that the data are normally distributed, and remind you that it would be normal to plot out the data to look for any odd results and get a 'feel' for your results.

Place the data into a table and use a scientific calculator (if you have one) to calculate the mean, the standard deviation, the variance, the sum of the cases and the sum of the cases squared.

Now we need to make sure that the variances of our sample groups are not significantly different (see criterion 4 on p.127). To do this, select the largest and smallest variances and perform an F test as shown in Chapter 10.

There is no significant difference in the variances so we can proceed with the test.

Step 1: calculate a correction factor (CF) this makes the calculations a little quicker.

$$CF = \frac{(\Sigma x_{tot})^2}{n_{tot}} = \frac{(519.70)^2}{30} = \frac{270088.09}{30} = 9002.93$$

Step 2: calculate the sums of squares (SS) for the whole sample.

$$SS_{tot} = \Sigma x^2_{tot} - CF = 10036.9 - 9002.9 = 1034$$

Step 3: calculate the between groups sums of squares.

$$SS_{between} = \frac{(\Sigma x_{GP1})^2}{n_{GP1}} + \frac{(\Sigma x_{GP2})^2}{n_{GP2}} + \frac{(\Sigma x_{GP3})^2}{n_{GP3}} - CF$$

$$SS_{between} = \frac{19016.4}{10} + \frac{51619.8}{10} + \frac{23890.8}{10} - CF$$

$$SS_{between} = 1901.6 + 5161.9 + 2389.1 - 9002.93$$

$$SS_{between} = 449.67$$

Step 4: calculate within groups sums of squares. A short cut can be used here because we know that the between-groups' and within-groups' SS must add up to the total.

$$SS_{total} = SS_{between} - SS_{within}$$

SO

$$SS_{within} = SS_{total} - SS_{between}$$

$$584.33 = 1034 - 449.67$$

If you are forced to do ANOVAs by hand it's probably best to calculate both the within-group and between-group SS by long hand as this will allow you to check your maths.

Step 5: determine the degrees of freedom for both the within and between groups following the following rules:

$$\text{d.f. for SS}_{between} = \text{number of groups} - 1$$

(In this example 3 – 1 = 2)

$$\text{d.f. for SS}_{within} = \text{total number of cases} - \text{the number of groups}$$

(In this example 30 – 3 = 27)

$$\text{d.f. for SS}_{total} = \text{d.f. SS}_{between} + \text{SS}_{within}$$

Step 6: calculate the variances for both the between and the within sums of squares:

$$S^2 \text{ between} = \frac{SS_{between}}{d.f._{between}} = \frac{449.67}{2} = 224.83$$

$$S^2 \text{ within} = \frac{SS_{within}}{d.f._{within}} = \frac{584.33}{27} = 21.64$$

Step 7 calculate F

$$F = \frac{Variance\ between\ groups}{Variance\ within\ groups} = \frac{224.83}{21.64} = 10.38$$

Step 7: it is normal for the results from an ANOVA to be put in a table laid out in a standard format like the one below. The results of ANOVAs performed using statistical packages are often presented in such tables.

TABLE 13.5

Source of variation	Sums of squares	d.f.	Variance	F
Between groups	449.67	2	224.83	10.38
Within groups	584.33	27	21.64	
Total	1034	29		

An alternative would be the following:

TABLE 13.6

Source of variation	Sums of squares	d.f.	Mean Squares	
Between Groups	449.67	2	224.83	10.38
Error	584.33	27	21.64	
Total	1034	29		

Step 8: look up the value of F in the appropriate statistical table (Appendix 3, Table 1). Note the variance between groups should always be on top, and be larger than the within-group variance. If the between group's variance is less than the within group's variance the null hypothesis is automatically accepted.

The value of 10.38 is significant at the $P < 0.01$ level and so we can reject the null hypothesis and say that the difference between the groups is significant. We would express this result by saying that there was a significant difference between the three treatment groups (ANOVA $F_{2,27}$ = 10.38 n = 30 P<0.01.). Unlike the t test we also give the degrees of freedom for both within and between groups. They are given as a subscript to the F statistic.

Box 13.7 Performing an ANOVA

1. Using the data from the Symphadiol study presented in Chapter 5, perform an ANOVA on the four experimental treatments.
2. Are the means significantly different?
3. Did you look at plots of the data?
4. What do you conclude?

Contrasting the means

You may have noted that there is a slight problem with the ANOVA in that whilst we can say that there is a significant difference between the sample groups, we can't say which groups are different from each other and which are not. Thus, in the first example we do not know if both exercise regimes are different from the control, or if they are different from each other, etc. Fortunately, we can do follow-up tests that allow us to determine which sample groups are significantly different from each other.

For those using computer packages there are a range of these follow-up test options with an assortment of names. The only one of these to avoid is the least significant difference test, as you will make the same error as if you did multiple t tests. The most conservative (tends towards a type II error) is the Scheffe's test. The least conservative (tends towards a type I error) is Duncan's multiple range test.

We will look at how one of these tests is calculated, namely the Tukey test. You only need to do this test if the result of your ANOVA test is significant.

Example from the literature 13.1 One-way analysis of variance

Do staffing levels predict missed care delivery? The relationship between staffing levels and care delivery is never far from health care professionals' and managers' minds. Kalisch et al. (2011) studied the relationship between staffing levels and care omission across 110

(Continued)

(Continued)

care units. Their study focused on nursing care. In total it had 4,288 participants. The study is quite complex, in that the authors had to work with and analyse a large number of variables. The main body of the work uses correlation (see Chapter 17). Not surprisingly they found a significant relationship between occurrences of care being omitted and level of staffing. They used one-way analysis of variance to determine if there were also significant differences in the level of omissions that could be attributed to type of unit. You can read all about it at: http://intqhc.oxfordjournals.org/content/23/3/302.full.pdf.

Tukey test

Step 1: first compute a test statistic called T.

$$T = (q) \times \sqrt{\frac{\text{Within groups mean squares}}{n}}$$

You know the *within group's mean squares* and can find it in your previous calculations. You can find q only by consulting a table showing the probability distribution of q. To find q you need to know the d.f. for the within group's variance (called v in most statistical tables) and the number of sample groups (called k in most statistical tables).

In our example: $T = (2.90) \times \sqrt{\dfrac{21.64}{10}}$ = 2.90 × 1.47 = 4.26

Step 2: for each group mean compute the difference between it and each other group mean. You could use a table like Table 13.7.

TABLE 13.7 Comparing means after an ANOVA test

Group means	Group 1: 13.79	Group 2: 22.72	Group 3: 15.46
Group 1: 13.79		9.05	1.67
Group 2: 22.72			7.26
Group 3: 15.46			

Step 3: compare the difference between each pair of means to the value of T. If the difference is larger then the difference between the two means is significant.

Box 13.8 Now, think about what you can conclude from this study

1. Which means are significantly different from each other?
2. What do you conclude? Is the conclusion different now that you have contrasted the means?
3. Would you make any recommendations based on the outcome of this study?

Example from the literature 13.2: One-way analysis of variance 2

Measuring the quality of care other than by means of direct patient outcomes is becoming a more widely used practice. One such measure is patient satisfaction. In a paper by Zebiene et al. (2004) the factors that influence patient satisfaction with primary care consultations in Lithuania are examined. The authors follow a method first used in a study published in the UK. Repeating studies in different contexts not only helps practitioners understand a phenomenon in a particular country, but also helps practitioners understand the potential viewpoints and perceptions of individuals from differing cultural backgrounds. The Zebiene et al. (2004) study uses one-way ANOVA to examine which variables related to 'patient expectations' influence whether or not patients are satisfied with their consultations. The study concludes that in the population studied the most important expectation that determined satisfaction was 'understanding and explanation', then 'emotional support'. Interestingly, 'getting information' was not considered to be as important as these other two factors. This paper outlines in considerable detail the analysis of the questionnaire that was used. It can be found at: http://intqhc.oxfordjournals.org/content/16/1/83.full?sid=6819f706-9f89-4eb5-adb7-47f44f16255c.

Independence

We said at the start of this chapter that for an ANOVA to be suitable the individual cases must be independent. What does this mean?

Independence means that there should be no way that the measurements taken from one individual or object can interfere with or be affected by those taken from other objects or individuals within a study.

For example, if you were issuing a questionnaire to two groups of people and it was possible that the two groups could talk to each other to discuss the questions, clearly here the samples would not be independent.

> ## Box 13.9
>
> 1. Using the results from the exercise in Box 13.5, perform a Tukey test.
> 2. Which means are significantly different from each other?
> 3. What do you conclude? Is the conclusion different now that you have contrasted the means?
> 4. Would you make any recommendations based on the outcome of this study?

Of course in some cases sample groups may contain the same individuals, particularly when you are following the response of individuals to a treatment. Here you must opt for a repeat measure design.

Repeat measure design of ANOVA

The repeat measure design should be used in any study where the same individual is tested more than once. It is analogous to the paired t test. These tests are also known as within-group tests. We will look at the within-group one-way ANOVA.

For this test we will simply look at the theory and at an ANOVA table. Worked examples can be found in texts such as Kerr et al. (2002).

If you design an experiment such that you follow a number of individuals, it stands to reason that you will have less variation caused by sampling error between the groups. Because you are using the same individuals in each sample group, the error between them is the same no matter which sampling group they are actually in. There will still be, of course, error due to intra-individual variation and random factors. (If there was no sampling error there would be much less need for statistics!)

> The sampling unit does not have to be a person, but the measurement must be made on the same object more than twice.

As you have less sampling error to deal with, you can use a smaller sample size; this is a major advantage of repeat measure experimental designs. If you just used a 'normal' ANOVA you would end up overestimating the between group's error and so be more likely to produce a type II error.

An example of a repeat measure design is shown in Table 13.8. It represents the diastolic blood pressure of four men, who have been given a regime of exercise to follow as part of a treatment for mild hypertension. Each participant was measured at the start of the exercise programme and at three and six weeks after the start.

TABLE 13.8 Diastolic blood pressure of four men aged between fifty-six and fifty-eight at the start of and during a prescribed exercise regime

Individual	At start	After 3 weeks	After 6 weeks
1	92	89	85
2	94	87	84
3	90	92	90
4	97	96	92

Variability within a group

Reduced between group

To take account of this reduced between-group error, the calculation of F is slightly altered, so that the error due to difference in the individuals is not taken into account when we compare the groups. To do this, the within group's error is divided into two components: that due to the individuals, called the sums of squares of the subjects, and sums of squares of the residual variation.

In other words:

$$SS_{within\ Groups} = SS_{Subjects} + SS_{Residual}$$

If we can determine the $SS_{Subjects}$ then we can remove it, and the $SS_{Within\ Groups}$ we used in the first ANOVA described will be substituted by the term $SS_{Residual}$

Fortunately we are able to compute $SS_{Subjects}$ and therefore perform a repeat measures ANOVA. However, we will not detail its calculation here.

When a repeat measures design is computed the ANOVA table will look like the one in Table 13.9. This ANOVA has been generated for the data presented in Table 13.8.

TABLE 13.9

Source of variation	Sums of squares	d.f.	Mean squares	F
Between groups	61.17	2	30.58	5.58
Residual error	32.83	6	5.47	

Again, you now must look to see if F is significant. We have assumed that you will be using a computer package. You will see that P will be reported as 0.043, in other words, P < 0.05, so the difference is significant.

If you have used a computer package you may well see reference to a phenomenon called sphericity. Sphericity, in the statistical sense, is an assumption that the variance of the differences between the experimental groups is not different. For most repeat measures designs ANOVAs we must assume sphericity and computer packages will perform a test of this assumption.

Having read this chapter and completed the exercises, you should be familiar with the follow ideas and concepts:

- when to perform a one-way ANOVA;
- when to use a repeat measure design one-way ANOVA;
- how to perform a one-way ANOVA;

- the rules that restrict the use of the ANOVA;
- how to contrast the means following a one-way ANOVA.

1. Using the data from the study of Symphadiol given in Chapter 5, plot a histogram using the descriptive statistics for group 1 (control), group 2, group 3 and group 4.
2. Plot a graph comparing these data and show the SEs.
3. State the hypothesis of the experiment.
4. State the statistical and null hypotheses.
5. Perform an appropriate statistical test(s): (a) by hand; (b) using a computer package.
6. Compare the results: which approach do you prefer and why?
7. What can you conclude about the impact of Symphadiol?
8. Collect a suitable data set of your own to perform an ANOVA. Remember the restrictions of this technique.

14

Not normal

Areas of learning covered in this chapter

- How do I know if my data are normally distributed?
- What are my options if my data are not normally distributed?
- When should I and how can I transform data?
- What is the Poisson distribution and why is it important?

In the chapters on comparing differences, you will have seen that most of the tests require your data set to be normally distributed, or at least not significantly different from normal (Chapter 11). This chapter seeks to address two problems: how do I know if my data are significantly different from normal and what do I do if they are?

If you looked at the chapter on *t* tests (Chapter 12) you will see that sometimes because the data set is small you have to rely on an assumption that the data set will be normally distributed, you can do this because variables recorded on particular measurement scales tend to be normally distributed, this is the case for example with most measures of human growth.

Similarly, other data such as percentages or counts of things you can probably say won't be normal. But what if you are unsure? What do you do then?

Of course, the first thing you should do is plot your data as a frequency histogram; if your data set is of thirty or more cases and your plot doesn't look normally distributed then you can safely assume that it isn't. But what if after doing your plot you're still unsure? In this case, you need to perform a statistical test, a test to tell you whether or not your data are significantly different from normal.

If you find that your data are *not* normally distributed you have two options: either transform the data, such that a parametric test is suitable, or use a **non-parametric** alternative (Chapter 15). You will want to use parametric tests if you can because they are more robust and powerful than the non-parametric alternative. Parametric tests are based on probability distributions, while non-parametric tests are not.

If you are using a computer, there are several easily accessible tests available. We shall discuss some of these options.

Box 14.1

What do the terms **skew** and **kurtosis** refer to?

If you don't have a statistical package available, you will probably want to use a test called the chi-square for goodness of fit. If on the other hand, you do have access to a statistics package then something like the Kolmogorov-Smirnov (KS) test, the Cochran's test or tests for skewness and kurtosis will probably be more straightforward. Do not ignore the goodness of fit test, as it is useful, particularly when looking to see is data fit other distribution types.

Test for normality

Both the KS test and the Cochran's test compare the tested distribution against standards. These tests produce a test statistic and like any other (x in the case of the Cochran's test and y in the case of the KS test) if the test statistic exceeds the critical value then your distribution is significantly different from normal. Most computer packages will report the test statistic and calculate a P value. All you need to do is spot if the P value is less than $P = 0.05$. If it is, then your distribution is significantly different from normal.

Box 14.2   Test procedure for kurtosis and skewness

A test can be performed similar to the z test to determine if a distribution is significantly skewed or shows significant kurtosis. For any given frequency distribution a z score (termed z_{skew} or $z_{kurtosis}$) for both skewness and kurtosis can be calculated. If either of these values exceeds 1.96, then the distribution in question can be said to differ significantly from normal. You then have two options: either transform your data to make it normal or use a non-parametric test (see Chapter 15).

Tests for skewness and kurtosis, on the other hand, can be used to determine if your distribution is significantly kurtosed or skewed. They take each of these measures one at a time.

Goodness of fit

The goodness of fit test that we will describe is based on the chi-square test for homogeneity described in Chapter 16. Many statistics texts recommend using the G-test instead of the chi-square, as it is more reliable. However, here we will stick to the chi-square as few computer programs support the G-test and we discuss the chi-square test elsewhere in this book. For a detailed discussion of the G-test, see Sokal and Rohlf (2012).

A goodness of fit test compares the distribution of numbers in a sample against a model distribution. If we are testing to see if your distribution is normal then the model distribution will be the normal distribution.

> **A warning**
>
> If you are doing your statistics by hand, do think twice about using a goodness of fit test to see if a normal distribution is appropriate. The process takes time and is tedious. Instead you could plot out your data and see if the data look normal. In addition you could estimate if 70 per cent of the cases lie within the bounds of the mean ± 1 SD.
>
> If your work is for publication it is likely, however, that some sort of test for normality will be required. An alternative would be to opt to use a non-parametric test that does not make assumptions about the distribution of the data.

The goodness of fit test can be used to test if your data fit any particular distribution. Thus, they can be used to see if data fit other theoretical population such as the **Poisson** or the binomial distributions.

For a goodness of fit test, we regard the sampled data as the 'observed data' and the model distribution as the 'expected'. We are testing to see if the observed frequency matches that predicted by the model distribution. For each observed case it is possible to predict how often it should occur theoretically and compare it to how often it actually does. Comparing observed results against expected results is the essence of the chi-square test.

For the normal distribution, the model equation that is used to Poisson the frequency for any given case (x) is shown below.

$$y = \frac{1}{\sigma\sqrt{(2\Pi)}} e^{-\left[(x-\mu)^2/2\sigma^2\right]}$$

In this equation, there are two constants (values that don't change): e and pi; the value of e is 2.71 and that of Π, 3.1417. x stands for the value of a particular case, μ stands for the population mean and σ for the population SD. Of course, because more often than not we are dealing with samples of populations we have to use $\bar{x}$ and s as estimates of μ and s. This gives rise to a slight problem in that we are trying to establish a model normal distribution, and in order to do that we need to be reasonably sure that our measures of $\bar{x}$ and s are reasonable estimates of μ and s. For this to be true, we need to have a *sample size more than 30*.

The chi-square bit

We can predict 'expected' from our model distribution, and as we have our own observed data we are in a position to perform a χ^2 (chi-square) test (Chapter 17). The formula for a χ^2 is as follows:

$$\chi^2 = \Sigma \frac{(O-E)^2}{E}$$

The test statistic is χ, O stands for observed and E expected. Σ of course stands for sum of. What do we sum? We sum each occurrence where we can compare an observed with an expected result.

An example

Janet Thompson is doing a small research project looking at the number of visits made to a walk-in treatment centre by different sections of the community. She uses a period of a week as her sampling unit and wants to compare the frequency of visits of white, Afro-Caribbean and Bangladeshi women. She suspects that as her data are counts of things her data samples may not be normally distributed. However, she wants to use parametric statistics, as she knows that these are more powerful and robust than the non-parametric alternatives.

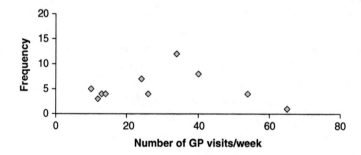

FIGURE 14.1 Frequency distribution of visits made to a walk-in treatment centre by Afro-Caribbean women

   She plots each of her cases. We will concentrate on the data for the Afro-Caribbean women. Are these data normally distributed? Looking at the graph we can say that the graph does seem a little skewed and there are more points below the mean than above it. The mean of the data is 31.7 and the standard deviation is 13.89, thus the variance (SD squared) is much larger than the mean and suggests that these data are positively skewed.

Box 14.3

Look back at Chapter 6 to see how to plot a frequency histogram.

TABLE 14.1 Calculating the standard deviation (s) and mean from a frequency table

No. of visits (x)	Frequency of visits(f)	Frequency of number of visits (fx)	$(x-\bar{x})^2$	$f(x-\bar{x})^2$
34	12	408	31.7	381.0
12	3	36	267.8	803.5
65	1	65	1342.1	1342.1
13	4	52	236.1	944.4
10	5	50	337.3	1686.4
54	4	216	657.1	2628.5
24	7	168	19.1	133.4
40	8	320	135.3	1082.9
26	4	104	5.6	22.4
14	4	56	206.4	825.5
	n = 52	$\Sigma fx = 1475$	$\bar{x} = \Sigma fx/n = 28.4$	$\Sigma f(x-\bar{x})^2 = 9850.1$
				s = 13.90

When you have formulated your data into a frequency table, a quick method of calculating the mean can be seen in Table 14.1. The standard deviation can be calculated as below:

$$s = \sqrt{\frac{\Sigma f(x-\bar{x})^2}{n-1}}$$

Now that you know the standard deviation, enter the figures into the equation that will predict the frequency of any case for a given mean and standard deviation if the numbers are drawn from a normal distribution. For our data the actual frequencies are given below.

Note that you do not convert the actual values into percentages. To obtain the expected frequencies you must multiply the predicted frequency for each value of x by n. Notice how low the predicted values are compared to the expected ones.

TABLE 14.2 The observed and expected (as predicted by the normal distribution) frequency of visits to a walk-in treatment centre by Afro-Caribbean women. The sample mean is 28.4 and the standard deviation 13.9

Number of visits	10	12	13	14	24	26	34	40	54	65
Actual frequency of that number of visits	5	3	4	4	7	4	12	8	4	1
Expected frequency	1	1	1	1	1.5	1.5	1.5	1	0.5	0.5

Box 14.4

Why are the expected values so low?

You're now in a position to do the actual goodness of fit test. For each value of x, perform the equation:

$$\frac{(O-E)^2}{E}$$

For the first value, this will be $\frac{(5-1)^2}{1}$ which gives a value of 16.

Repeat this for each value of x, and then add together all the results. You should get:

$16 + 4 + 9 + 9 + 20.2 + 4.2 + 73.5 + 49 + 24.5 + 0.5 = 209.9$

i.e. $\chi^2 = 209.9$

As with most tests you now have to look this value up in a table using the appropriate degrees of freedom. The table is the χ^2 distribution table (Appendix 3, Table 4). The degrees of freedom to use are the number of values − 2 (in this case 10 − 2). So, we have eight degrees of freedom. The value in Table 4 for a level of significance of 0.05 is 15.51, therefore our value (being bigger than that in the table) indicates that the difference between the observed and the expected frequencies is significant and we can conclude that the distribution under investigation is significantly different from the normal distribution.

Box 14.5

Collect a sample of the shoe sizes of about thirty people. Determine whether this sample is distributed in a manner that is significantly different from normal.

Using goodness of fit tests with the Poisson distribution

Goodness of fit tests can be used to see if frequency distributions fit any theoretical mathematical distribution of numbers. One important distribution for those working in health care is the Poisson distribution. This is because it is a distribution that describes rare phenomena that occur in space or time randomly. For example, how many times does lightning strike per unit of time? We might want to ask whether or not the occurrence of violent events in hospital A&E units are randomly dispersed across all hospitals in an area or whether they are associated with something to do with that hospital. We might ask does a disease such as myeloid leukaemia occur randomly across a particular country or is it associated with some other phenomena such as the location? Because the Poisson distribution describes random distributions, we can use it to test if our data are randomly distributed or not. Test for a Poisson distribution if:

- your data represent rare phenomena;
- the data is composed of counts of things;
- the variance is quite similar to the mean.

The formula for predicting the probability of finding x number of occurrences of the rare phenomena in a given sample is:

$$P_{(x)} = e^{-\overline{X}} \cdot \frac{\overline{X}^x}{x!}$$

Who said life would be simple! By computer, it is possible to extract these values more easily. Most of the mathematical functions in the equation you have seen before with the exception of x!. The symbol ! means factorial. The factorial of 3 would be the product of 1 x 2 x 3 = 6. The factorial of 5 would be 1 x 2 x 3 x 4 x 5 = 120. The · is short hand for multiply; e is of course 2.71 (the base of the natural logarithm).

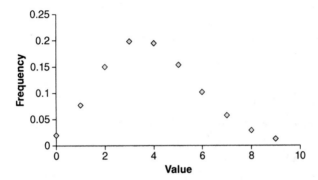

FIGURE 14.2 A Poisson distribution

So if $x = 3$ and the mean of your sample is 6:

$$P_{(3)} = e^{-6} \cdot \frac{6}{3!} = 0.045$$

In other words, if the phenomenon is randomly distributed then we have a 4.5 per cent chance of obtaining a value of value of 3.

We will use an example to demonstrate. Eastern Health Authority is concerned about recent outbreaks of MRSA in a number of its wards. It is believed that there may be some link between outbreaks in different wards in different hospitals. The infection control officers sample forty wards across their area and record the number of patients who have apparently contracted an MRSA infection whilst in hospital. They find the following frequencies of infection.

The average number of infections per ward is 3.75. As with the example from the normal distribution, you now use the mathematical model of the (Poisson) distribution to predict the expected frequency for this mean. As before, having found the expected frequency you can now perform a χ-square test for goodness of fit.

In this case $\chi^2 = 9.22$. The degrees of freedom = the number of values −2 so in this case we have 10−2 = 8. With eight degrees of freedom the critical value in the χ^2 distribution table is 15.51 at $P = 0.05$. As our calculated value of χ^2 is less than 15.51 we can say that there is no significant

TABLE 14.3   The observed and expected frequencies (as predicted by the Poisson distribution) of the number of MRSA-infected patients across wards in the eastern region

Number of infected patients	O	1	2	3	4	5	6	7	8	9
Frequency	3	3	5	6	6	5	3	2	2	1
Expected frequency	0.7	3.0	6.0	7.9	7.8	6.2	4.1	2.3	1.1	0.5

difference between the observed values and those predicted by the Poisson distribution. We can therefore conclude that the occurrences of MSRA in the eastern region show a distribution that is not significantly different from random.

Transforming

If you have tested your data and they are not normal, the rest of this chapter devotes itself to what to do next.

What is a transformation?

Simply put, a **transformation** is where we alter the distribution of a set of data by applying a mathematical function to each case. We might, for example, square root each case. If this sounds like fiddling your data it isn't. Transformations have been used for many years and their soundness has been tested over many years. For most of the common deviations from the normal distribution, there is a standard transformation.

Here we will describe three types of transformation: the logarithmic, the arcsine and the square root. These are probably the most common.

The logarithmic transformation

We use a logarithmic (log.) transformation where it is noticed that the variance of the samples increases with the mean, where the data are clumped (there is a large frequency of cases against just one or two values) and where the frequency distribution is skewed to the right.

To perform a log. transformation, simply log all the cases. You then perform the appropriate statistical test on the logged data. Having logged the data, you should of course check that the new distribution isn't significantly different from normal. Do not forget that the standard error and confidence limits rely on the data set being normal. If you want to quote these values you must first calculate the values using the transformed data, and then antilog the values to obtain quotable meaningful figures. With all transformations, you must reverse the transformation in order to report means, SEs and confidence limits.

Box 14.6

When should you quote a SE?

If your data are composed of counts of something and you have a lot of zeros try using log (x + 1), i.e. add one to each case and then log the result.

The arcsine transformation

This transformation is useful for data that have been recorded as percentages or proportions. It is sometimes called the angular transformation.

The formula for the arcsine transformation is:

$$TV = \arcsin \sqrt{p}$$

where *TV* stands for the transformed value and *P* for a proportion.

If the cases of your data have been measured as proportion (a percentage is simply a special type of proportion: divide by 100 and then proceed) then every case represents a *P*. If the cases in your sample fall in the range of 0.30 – 0.70 (30–70 per cent) there is no need to transform these data.

In order to perform an arcsine transformation first square root all your samples then obtain the angle of the sine of the resultant. On calculators, use the inverse sine (sin-[1]key). The answer should be expressed in degrees.

To convert back to normal values, again take each transformed value, find its sine and square this value.

The square root transformation

If your samples are Poisson distributed (the variance is similar to the mean) then you will need to use the square root transformation. As the name of this transformation suggests, each case should be square rooted, then the statistical test applied. Values can be squared to report the mean SE and confidence limits. If the data contains zeros, rather than take the square root take the square root of (x + 0.5), i.e. add 0.5 to each case then square root it.

For a thorough discussion of transformations, see Sokal and Rohlf (2012).

Having read this chapter and completed the exercises, you should be familiar with the following ideas and concepts:

- why transformations are used;
- how to use a c-square test for goodness of fit test;
- the Poisson distribution;
- the application of the logarithmic, arcsine and square root transformations.

1. Using the data on age from the questionnaire (Chapter 5), perform an appropriate test to see if these data are normally distributed. Note this is difficult without the help of a statistical package.
2. What type of distribution does the variable 'number of partners' have? Can you transform these data to make them follow a normal distribution? Why might you want to?

15

Non-parametric tests

Areas of learning covered in this chapter

- What are non-parametric tests?
- When should non-parametric tests be used?
- What types of basic non-parametric test are there?

Up until now, we have described tests that are known as parametric tests. These tests rely on the data being distributed in a certain way (quite often, normally). Parametric tests are thought to be the most powerful tests as they also allow very in-depth statistical interrogation and testing of data. Unfortunately, a substantial amount of the data we collect in relation to health care research is not normally distributed and our ability to transform such data to a normal distribution is limited (see Chapter 14). This chapter will introduce a range of tests that do not rely on the data conforming to a certain distribution. As such they can be used with data that are not normally distributed, known as non-parametric tests. We have already come across one group of non-parametric tests, those that use the χ^2 statistic. This chapter will describe some of the non-parametric tests that are analogous to the parametric tests described in this book.

Health care research often involves us working as social scientists. We are often involved in collecting a wide range of qualitative data, and we are often interested in variables that are measured on the ordinal scale (e.g. perceived amount of pain, anxiety state) or nominal scale (e.g. profession, type of education, housing type, ethnic group). Such variables are less likely to be normally distributed and therefore you will need to be familiar with non-parametric tests.

When to use non-parametric tests

Non-parametric tests should be used when the data does not conform to the conditions required for a parametric test.

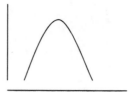

FIGURE 15.1   Normal distribution

Normally when we consider population distributions, we use such parameters as the mean or standard deviation. This is fine if the distribution of your data is normal.

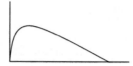

FIGURE 15.2   Skewed distribution

However, in distributions that are not normally distributed (Figure 15.1) but skewed (Figure 15.2) or distributed in some other way (see Chapter 6) and the mean is not an appropriate descriptive test to use (see Chapter 6), then a non-parametric test is probably more appropriate.

Non-parametric tests can also be used on small samples. We have described a parametric test, the student's *t* test that is appropriate for small samples. If, however, you are unsure that the data collected will conform to a normal distribution and your sample is small then it is safer to opt for a non-parametric test.

Non-parametric tests are normally used for data collected using the ordinal and nominal scales of measurement. However, they can also be used for interval and ratio measurements where the distribution does not conform to normality.

Non-parametric tests are not based on distributions, but on exact probabilities; they do not use the mean, and are more likely to be based on comparing the extent to which data deviates from the median. As such, when using non-parametric tests it is more appropriate to quote the median.

Box 15.1   Choice of statistic

Review three or four research articles that use a statistical approach:

1. See if you can spot the type of statistic used (parametric or non-parametric).
2. Discuss the justification used for that particular choice.

Finally, non-parametric tests can be conducted on data from subjects that have not been randomly selected from the population from which they derive. In health care research, it can be difficult to achieve a **random sample** because samples are often convenience based and as such not randomly drawn from the population. Care must be taken, however, to bear this in mind when interpreting the results.

Box 15.2   Difference between parametric and non-parametric tests

Non-parametric

- can be used on ordinal and nominal scale data (although also on interval and ratio scale);
- can be used on small samples;
- can be used on data that are not normally distributed;
- can be used where the samples are not selected randomly;
- have less power than the equivalent parametric test.

Parametric

- used mainly on interval and ratio scale data;
- tend to need larger samples;
- data should fit a particular distribution, the data can be transformed to that distribution;
- samples should be drawn randomly from the population;
- more powerful than non-parametric equivalent.

The principle behind using a non-parametric procedure as a statistical test is the same as for parametric procedures. You form a hypothesis, gather your data, subject that data to the appropriate statistical equations (depending on the test chosen), produce a test statistic and, finally, see if your result is statistically significant by looking the result up in statistical tables using the appropriate degrees of freedom. Remember we perform statistical tests so that we know that if we find a difference or a relationship we can be sure it did not arise by chance.

Ranking data

Many non-parametric tests involve ranking the data. In the next section we explore this process.

Ranking is simply a way of placing all the cases in order. For example, two groups of students watched a health promotion video and valued it out of ten, with 1 = poor and 10 = excellent. The students from school A gave the video values of 3, 5, 6 and 6. The pupils from school B gave it 1, 3, 6, 8. To rank these scores first place all the numbers together in numerical order as follows:

1, 3, 3, 5, 6, 6, 6, 8

We then assign each a number that corresponds to its position in the original numerical line-up (order). We can then assign a rank to each score. If in your data sets all the scores (values) just occur once then the rank will correspond to the order. The scores will then be known as values.

TABLE 15.1 Values that school children gave to a health promotion video The values have been ordered and then ranked

Values	1	3	3	5	6	6	6	8
Order	1	2	3	4	5	6	7	8
Rank	1	2.5	2.5	4	6	6	6	8

Unfortunately, in our example, as is common in most studies, some of our values occur more than once and as such we need to take this into account when determining rank.

Determining rank score

To do this, where a score (value) occurs more than once we add the order of those values together and divide by the number of times that the particular score (value) occurs. The result becomes the rank for that score (value).

Box 15.3 Practice ranking

Ask twelve friends or colleagues to score on a scale of 1–10 the quality of the last meal that they bought. Ask another group to score on the same scale the last meal they made for themselves.
   Order and rank each set of values

In the example above (Table 15.1), the value 3 occurs twice and occupies two positions in the order, namely 2 and 3. To calculate rank we thus add 2 and 3 together, and divide by the number of times the value 3 occurs (2). Thus, the rank for the value 3 is 2.5. Repeating this for the other value where there is another tie (for the value 6), you get the ranks as shown in Table 15.1

The tests

Test for difference in two independent or unrelated samples: a substitute for the student's t test and the z test.

The Mann–Whitney U test is a non-parametric test for differences in the **median** of two independent samples. As with the t test, independent means that the groups are not connected. You must have a set of data with regards to a parameter from one group of participants or objects and a second set from a different group.

TABLE 15.2 The attitude scores of people to the siting of an asylum centre in the vicinity of their village (1 = very positive, 10 = very negative)

West Village	East Village
1	2
2	3
2	3
3	5
5	6
5	8
6	8
6	9
7	9
7	10
7	
8	

The Mann–Whitney U test calculates the test statistic U. This statistic is then looked up in the appropriate statistical table and its significance determined. As with most statistical tests we start with a hypothesis. In the example below, social worker Amber Smith has measured the attitude of members of the public to having a reception centre for asylum seekers located in the vicinity of their village. She has scored attitude on a 1–10 scale with 1 being very positive and 10 very negative. She hypothesized before undertaking her study that people from West village would have a more negative attitude as this village is more wealthy and people would be more concerned about the impact of the centre on property prices. Amber Smith is concerned that the centre is located in a site that is sensitive to the views of the community as this will influence both the social well-being of the asylum seekers and the villagers. The results of her study are shown in Table 15.2. The formula of the Mann–Whitney U test is as follows:

$$U_1 = n_1 \times n_2 + \frac{n_2(n_2 + 1)}{2} - R_2$$

$$U_2 = n_1 \times n_2 + \frac{n_1(n_1 + 1)}{2} - R_1$$

You can no doubt see that two values of U are calculated, U_1 and U_2. You will see later how these two values are used. n_1 stands for the sample size of the first sample and n_2 that of the second, R_1 the sum of the ranks from the first sample and R_2 the sum of the ranks from the second.

Remember that to rank the data, both sets have to be arranged together; do not rank groups separately.

Step 1: rank the data (Table 15.3). Note we have included an indication as to which village each value and rank came from. Also, note that several of the values are repeated.

TABLE 15.3

Village	W	W	W	E	W	E	E	W	W	E	W	W	E	W	W	W	W	E	E	E	E	E
Value	1	2	2	2	3	3	3	5	5	5	6	6	6	7	7	7	8	8	8	9	9	10
Order	1	2	3	4	5	6	7	8	9	10	11	12	13	14	15	16	17	18	19	20	21	22
Rank	1	3	3	3	6	6	6	9	9	9	12	12	12	15	15	15	18	18	18	21.5	21.5	22

Step 2: separate out the ranks of each sample (Table 15.4).

TABLE 15.4

Village	W	W	W		W			W	W		W	W					W	W	W	W
Rank	1	3	3		6			9	9		12	12					15	15	15	18

Village			E		E	E		E		E					E	E	E	E	E
Rank			3		6	6		9		12					18	18	21.5	21.5	22

Step 3: sum the ranks for each sample (village). Sum of ranks for West village (ΣR_1) = 1 + 3 + 3 + 6 + 9 + 9 + 12 + 12 + 15 + 15 + 15 + 18 = 118. Sum of ranks for East village (ΣR_2) =137.

Step 4: load the values into the first equation.

$$U_1 = 12 \times 10 + \frac{10(10+1)}{2} - 137$$

$$U_1 = 120 + \frac{110}{2} - 137$$

$$U_1 = 120 + 55 - 137$$

$$U_i = 38$$

Step 5: repeat for the second equation.

$$U_2 = n_1 \times n_2 + \frac{n_1(n_1+1)}{2} - R_1$$

$$U_2 = 12 \times 10 + \frac{12(12+1)}{2} - 118$$

$$U_2 = 120 + 78 - 118$$

$$U_2 = 80$$

So, $U_1 = 38$ and $U_2 = 80$. In the Mann–Whitney U test we are interested in the smallest value only. Therefore for the purposes of this test $U = 38$.

Box 15.4 A new descriptive statistic?

The sum of the ranks provides us with a descriptive of how different the two villages' attitude to the asylum centre is. We can see that the sum of the ranks is 118 for West village and for East village, it is 137. This indicates that West village has lower scores. If the two populations did not differ very much you would expect the scores to be similar and therefore not to be significantly different. The sum of ranks can be a useful descriptive statistic to present as it provides a greater level of precision than the median.

We now must look this value up in the table of Mann–Whitney U test values (Appendix 3, Table 6), using the sample sizes of 10 and 12 (as these were the sample sizes from the two villages). The critical value from the table is 29. As our value is *greater* than this, we are unable to reject the null hypothesis. Note this is the only test we have described so far in this book, where if the critical value is exceeded the null hypothesis is not rejected. Amber Smith concludes that there is no significant difference in the attitudes of the two villages towards the asylum centre.

Box 15.5 Finding the difference

For the data you obtained for the exercise in Box 15.3 perform a Mann–Whitney U test to see if there is a difference in the medians of the values.
What difficulties can you see in using scores of this nature?

You will notice that the Mann–Whitney U table does not exceed twenty. At sample sizes above twenty the distribution of U begins to approximate to the normal distribution, and what this means in layman's terms is that the normal distribution should be used instead. To do this you must convert your U statistic to a t statistic using the following formula:

$$t = \frac{U - (n_1 \times n_2)/2}{\dfrac{n_1 x n_2 (n_1 + n_2 + 1)}{12}}$$

The calculated value of t can then be looked up in the t distribution tables.

Restrictions on the use of the Mann–Whitney *U* test

Conditions for the use of interval and ratio and ordinal scale data, as well as proportions, percentages and counts.

Samples or groups should come from data that has similar distributions, although they do not need to be the same.

If your ranked data contains a large number of ties, a correction needs to be made. This correction is given automatically on most statistical packages.

It can only be used to contrast two groups.

Example from the literature 15.1   Mann–Whitney *U* test

Different types of patients from similar sections of the population can sometimes end up in differing care settings. Bannister et al.'s (1998) study examined the characteristics of dementia suffers who entered residential care as opposed to those who did not. The Mann–Whitney *U* test was used extensively in this study to compare characteristics such as 'coping strategies' and severity of Parkinson's syndrome (see their Table 1). This study also used odds ratios and a more complex test called the logistic regression, which is not covered by this textbook. Bannister et al.'s study can be accessed at: http://her. oxfordjournals.org/content/13/1/47.full.pdf+html.

Tests for differences between two related samples: the Wilcoxon's two-sample test - a substitute for the paired *t* test

In the above example our two sets of data were not related – they were collected from two independent groups of villagers. There are many ways that data can be classified as related; for example, each person may be asked to evaluate two different forms of birth control. Consequently, each person provides two pieces of data that are considered related. Equally, people may be paired by similar characteristics or sets of parameters. Finally, there are before and after tests where once again one individual provides two pieces of data. In these cases, it is not possible to use the Mann–Whitney *U* test but instead the **Wilcoxon's test** can be used. The test statistic calculated in the Wilcoxon's test is called *T*.

In the next example, a manager of a general practice is evaluating the impact of an advanced practitioner training course on the perception of a group of patients of the quality of service delivered by the practice nurse. The manager decided to give a questionnaire to a group of ten patients who needed to visit the nurse on a regular basis. He asked the patients to complete the questionnaire before and after the nurse had attended the course. As the same patients were used the samples were related. As the measurement, in this case an evaluation of overall quality, was on the ordinal scale the manager selected the Wilcoxon's two-sample test.

TABLE 15.5 Patient scores of quality of service before and after the practice nurse had attended a training course

Patient	Before	After	Difference
1	2	8	−6
2	5	3	+2
3	6	5	+1
4	5	6	−1
5	9	4	+5
6	7	3	+4
7	8	1	+7
8	7	5	+2
9	6	3	+3
10	5	2	+3

TABLE 15.6 The differences in the scores of the pairs from Table 15.5, ordered and then ranked

Difference	+1	−1	+2	+2	+3	+3	+4	+5	−6	+7
Order	1	2	3	4	5	6	7	8	9	10
Rank	1.5	1.5	3.5	3.5	5.5	5.5	7	8	9	10

Once the data has again been entered into a table (see Table 15.5), subtract one column from the other. It does not matter which set of data you enter in which column. The first step is to calculate the differences between each of the pairs, in this case the result before and the result after the training.

The second step is to rank the differences using the same techniques as in the Mann–Whitney U test. When doing this, ignore any values where the difference = zero, and also use the absolute value of the difference, that is ignore the signs at this stage.

Step 3 is to sum the ranks where the difference has a negative sign, and then sum the ranks where the difference has a positive sign.

Sum of the negative difference ranks = 1.5 + 9 = 10.5

Sum of the positive difference ranks = 1.5 + 3.5 + 3.5 + 5.5 + 5.5 + 7 + 8 + 10 = 44.5

Whichever sum is the smaller is given the value T.

Therefore, in this case $T = 10.5$

Having found the test statistic we now need to establish a value that is equivalent to the degrees of freedom in other tests; this value is called N. To calculate the value of N count the numbers of pairs of scores but subtract any whose difference was 0. In this case there were no differences of 0, therefore $N = 10$

Using the table of critical values of T (Appendix 3, Table 7) by locating the row where $N = 10$, the critical value is 10. In the Wilcoxon's two-sample test if the test statistic is equal or smaller (as with the Mann–Whitney U test this is the opposite of most statistical tests) than the critical value then the result is significant. In this case a 10.5 is not significant at the P < 0.05 level whether it is a one-tailed test, or a two-tailed test.

Box 15.6   One- or two-tailed test

Using your judgement decide if this test should be a one- or two-tailed test. Discuss the reasons why you have reached this conclusion.

Restrictions on the use of the Wilcoxon's two-sample test

The Wilcoxon's test makes the assumption that the samples have been drawn from populations that have symmetrical distribution. In particular it should not be used where the distributions are skewed.

Example from the literature 15.2   The Wilcoxon's two-sample test

In 1998 Marsh and Kendrick investigated the influence of a training programme on the knowledge of a range of practitioners of injuries prevention. The focus of the work was injuries prevention to children and in the home. At the time home injuries were a significant cause of child mortality within the study area.

The study was relatively simple. The authors tested the knowledge of the participants before educational intervention and then afterwards. They had scores for the same individuals before and after the intervention and so a two-sample test was appropriate. The authors used a Likert-type scale that they summed together; such a process often produces data that is distributed normally. However, the authors decided to opt for the Wilcoxon two-sample test (which in this paper was given its alternative name of Wilcoxon matched-pairs signed rank test). They did not do any distribution test. The post-intervention questionnaires were issued three to four months after the intervention. You can read the study at: http://her.oxfordjournals.org/content/13/1/47.full.pdf+html.

Test for difference in more than two independent or unrelated samples: a substitute for the one-way analysis of variance.

The Kruskal–Wallis H test is a test of significance used when there are more than two independent samples and when alternative parametric tests cannot be used. It can be used with data measured on the ordinal, interval or ratio scales.

In a previous example, we compared the data from two villages with regard to their attitude towards the siting of an asylum centre, but what if we wanted to introduce a third sample, North Village? We could conduct three Mann-Whitney U tests as outlined below:

School A by B

School A by C

School B by C

The problem with this, however, is that there is an increased likelihood of producing a type I error (just the same situation as when we were to perform multiple *t* tests – see Chapter 13). A type I error is when the null hypothesis is rejected when it should be accepted. The Kruskal–Wallis test is the non-parametric version. It should be used where you have two or more samples or groups of data that are not normally distributed.

TABLE 15.7 The attitude scores of people to the siting of an asylum centre in the vicinity of their village (1 = very positive, 10 = very negative)

West Village	East Village	North Village
1	2	8
2	3	9
2	3	10
3	5	9
5	6	8
5	8	7
6	8	6
6	9	9
7	9	8
7	10	9
7		10
8		

The Kruskal–Wallis test is very similar to the Wilcoxon's test and also uses ranks. The test aims to determine if there are significant differences between the groups. It actually tests for a significant difference between the average ranks.

In the following example, Amber Smith has introduced a new village (North Village) into her sample, to analyse the data she needs to use a Kruskal–Wallis test.

As with the Wilcoxon's test the first step is to order and then rank the data (noting from which sample each of the ranks came from).

Remember to combine all the groups when ranking the data. Do not rank each group separately.

Having calculated the ranks, the next step is to calculate for each sample (Village) the sum of the ranks, the square of the sum of the ranks and R^2/n.

TABLE 15.8 The scores and ranks of the data presented in Table 15.8

West Village	Rank West Village	East Village	Rank East Village	North Village	Rank North Village
1	1	2	3	8	21.5
2	3	3	6	9	27.5
2	3	3	6	10	32
3	6	5	9	9	27.5
5	9	6	12.5	8	21.5
5	9	8	21.5	7	16.5
6	12.5	8	21.5	6	12.5
6	12.5	9	27.5	9	27.5
7	16.5	9	27.5	8	21.5
7	16.5	10	32	9	27.5
7	16.5			10	32
8	21.5				

TABLE 15.9 Statistical summary of the ranking data presented in Table 15.8

	West Village	East Village	North Village
Sample size (n)	12	10	11
Sum of ranks (ΣR)	127	166.5	295
ΣR^2	16129	27722	87025
$\Sigma R^2/n$	1344	2772	7911

Two more values that we need to know are N, the sum of the sample size (Σn), and also $\Sigma(\Sigma R^2/n)$, the sum of all the values in the final row of Table 15.9. In this case $N = 33$ and $\Sigma (\Sigma R^2/n) = 12027$

The next step is to plug your values into the equation that produces the test statistic that in this case is called H.

$$H = \left[\Sigma(R^2/n) \times \frac{12}{N(N+1)} \right] - 3(N+1)$$

$$H = \left[12027 \times \frac{12}{33 \times 32} \right] - 102$$

$$H = \left[12027 \times 0.011 \right] - 102$$

$$H = 30.29$$

Having found the test statistic K we now must look this up in the appropriate table, in this case it is the distribution of χ^2. As this test uses the χ^2 distribution to find the appropriate critical value, we must first calculate the degrees of freedom used. They are calculated by taking the number of samples (in this case 3, i.e. three villages) and subtracting 1. Therefore, in this example there are two degrees of freedom. At $P = 0.05$, the critical value is 5.99. The calculated value is *bigger* than this value, so in this case we *reject the null* hypothesis. In theory a correction should be made in the calculation of H where there are ties. However, in practice this makes very little difference to the overall result.

Box 15.7   Kruskal–Wallis test

Using the data you analysed in Box 15.5, ask another ten people to score the quality of the last meal that they ate. Use a Kruskal–Wallis test to determine if the difference in the three groups is significant.
   What potential problems can you see with this study?

Restrictions on the use of the Kruskal–Wallis test

If you are testing for differences between just three groups, you need to have data from at least five participants or objects for each group.

The data can be interval and ratio and ordinal scale data, as well as proportions, percentages and counts.

Correlation: a substitute test for the Pearson's correlation coefficient, the Spearman rank correlation

The Spearman rank correlation is a test that is used to determine the extent a change in one variable tends to be associated with a change in another. The correlation techniques we will look at seek to test for linear correlation, that is are the variables associated along a straight line continuum. Where one variable is associated with another in this way they are said to be correlated. The Spearman rank can be used with data collected on ordinal, ratio and interval scales. It is ideal for use where sample sizes are small (less than twenty).

When we perform a correlation, we not only ask if there is a correlation but we also want to know how strong the relationship is. The correlation test asks how strong is the relationship and is the correlation greater than could be expected by chance. To perform a correlation you must have measures of two different variables from the same participant or object.

In the following example, we have used data taken from Pittet et al. (2000) who investigated the effectiveness of a hospital-wide programme to improve compliance with hand hygiene. The aspect of this that we will look at is the relationship between the amount of alcohol hand-rub used per patient day and the incidence of hospital acquired MRSA. The study was based on a Swiss hospital.

TABLE 15.10   The relationship between alcohol hand-rub use and incidence of MSRA in a Swiss hospital

Year	Alcohol based hand-rub l/1000 patient days	New MRSA/100 admissions
1993	3.5	0.50
1994	4.1	0.60
1995	6.9	0.48
1996	9.5	0.32
1997	10.9	0.25
1998	15.4	0.26

The research question is, thus, is there a relationship between the amount of hand-rub used and the incidence of hospital acquired MRSA, the hypothesis being that as more hand-rub is used the incidence of MRSA should decrease. There are insufficient data here to perform a Pearson correlation (Chapter 17). In addition, it is unlikely that the measurement of MRSA per patient would come from a normal distribution, thus a Spearman rank correlation is appropriate for these data.

The Spearman rank correlation

As the name implies, the Spearman rank correlation involves ranking the data. In the case of the Spearman rank correlation, each variable is ranked separately, and the difference between the rank for each pair of variables for each participant or 'object' recorded. In our current example, the 'object' is a year.

TABLE 15.11   The data from Table 15.10, showing ranks and differences between the ranks

Year	Alcohol based hand-rub l/1000 patient days	Rank	New MRSA/100 admissions	Rank	Difference in ranks (d)	d²
1993	3.5	1	0.50	5	4	16
1994	4.1	2	0.60	6	4	16
1995	6.9	3	0.48	4	1	1
1996	9.5	4	0.32	3	1	1
1997	10.9	5	0.25	1	4	16
1998	15.4	6	0.26	2	4	16

We also need to calculate d^2 and Σd^2. In this case $\Sigma d^2 = 66$.

As normal, having done the basic calculation now plug the values into the appropriate equation to produce the test statistic, in this case the Spearman rank correlation coefficient or r_s. The equation is:

$$r_s = 1 - \frac{6 \times \Sigma d^2}{n^3 - n}$$

n in this case is 6, as we have six samples.

$$r_s = 1 - \frac{6 \times 66}{(6 \times 6 \times 6) - 6}$$

$$r_s = 1 - \frac{396}{210}$$

$$r_s = -0.88$$

In correlation, a value of 1 indicates a perfect positive relationship whilst a value of −1 indicates a perfect negative relationship, a value of 0 would indicate that there was no relationship (see Chapter 17). Our value of −0.88 indicates that the two variables are negatively correlated, meaning that as one variable increases (amount of hand-rub used) the other decreases (MRSA infection rate), but is this correlation statistically significant? As normal we turn to the appropriate statistical table (Appendix 3, Table 5). With a sample size of six, the critical value is 0.829 for a one-tailed test at $P < 0.05$. Thus there is a significant negative relationship between the amount of alcohol hand-rub used and the incidence of hospital acquired MRSA.

Restrictions on the use of the Spearman's rank correlation

As with all correlation techniques, a strong correlation does not mean that there is cause and effect.

Once the sample size exceeds thirty, the result obtained using either the Pearson correlation or the Spearman rank correlation will be similar.

If too many ranks are tied, error may be introduced into the calculation of the Spearman Rank Regression Correlation.

Example from the literature 15.3   Spearman's rank and Kruskal–Wallis test

Systemic sclerosis is a debilitating autoimmune disease that gives rise to microvascular injury and extensive fibrosis of the skin and internal organs. Nevertheless, people with systemic sclerosis are able to live productive lives. Sandqvist et al. (2010) in a classic descriptive correlation-based study sought to identify individual and work-related factors that influenced the ability of individuals to work and to examine the extent to which ability to work is linked to employment status, activities of daily life and quality of life.

The authors set themselves a complex task. They examined the relationship between the various variables largely using the Kruskal–Wallis test and Spearman's rank correlations. Kruskal–Wallis tests are used to examine the differences between level of work ability (three different levels) in relation to a range of social variables and disease variables. Many of these variables are measured using truncated and subjective scales and so are unlikely to be normally distributed. They used Spearman's rank correlations to examine the relationships between employment status, individual factors and work-related factors. The paper can be found at: http://rheumatology.oxfordjournals.org/content/early/2010/05/27/rheumatology.keq145.full.pdf.

Summary of tests

TABLE 15.12   Summary of tests

Name of test	Test is for	Number of samples/groups	Substitute for
Mann–Whitney U	Testing for difference in the medians of two unrelated/ independent samples.	2	t test
Wilcoxon	Testing for difference in the medians of two related samples/ paired samples.	2	paired t test
Kruskal-Wallis	Testing for difference in the medians of more than two unrelated/independent samples.	3 or more	one way ANOVA
Spearman rank	Test for correlations between two variables recorded from the same sampling unit.	1	Pearson's correlation

All these tests can be used for variables where the measurement is recorded on the ordinal, interval or ratio scales.

Having read this chapter and completed the exercises, you should be familiar with the following ideas and concepts:

- the difference between parametric and non-parametric tests;
- the types of data that can be investigated using basic non-parametric tests;

- the type of statistical question that can be asked using basic non-parametric tests;
- the Mann–Whitney U test;
- the Wilcoxon's test;
- the Kruskal–Wallis test;
- the Spearman rank correlation.

EXERCISES

1. Using the data from the walk-in centre questionnaire, perform an appropriate test to see if there is a difference between the number of sexual partners of individuals from the Asian and African ethnic groups. What explanations do you think there are for this relationship?
2. Repeat question 1 above, only this time include the individuals from the European ethnic group.
3. Is there a significant decrease in the number of sexual partners with age?

16

Tests for association: chi-square

Areas of learning covered in this chapter

- What are tests for association and chi-square tests?
- How are chi-square tests used?
- What types of restrictions are there on the use of chi-square tests?

Test for association

Sometimes when conducting studies we are interested in whether there is an association between two variables rather than a difference. For example, you may be interested to know if certain pathologies are associated with certain ethnic groups, knowing such information would help with the planning of health care services and the development of public health campaigns. An example of such associations is that between Afro-Caribbean communities and sickle cell anaemia and the association between cystic fibrosis and white Caucasian groups. When the association you are looking for involves data measured using the nominal scale it is normal to use chi-square tests.

Other types of association are where we find that a change in one variable tends to be associated with a change in another. For example, there is an association between age and occurrence of breast cancer. Sometimes we may find a decrease in one variable as another variable increases. For example, there is an association between increasing wealth and decreasing incidence of mental health problems. These types of associations are known as correlations. Correlations normally involve using data that has been measured on the ordinal, interval or ratio scales. In this chapter we will look at chi-square test and in Chapter 17 correlations.

The symbol for chi is c, thus the shorthand for chi-square is c^2. There are several forms of the c^2 test. They are, however, all based on the c^2 distribution and (although we use them to test for associations) are based on looking for a difference between what we expect to be the result and what we actually observed. Chi-square tests are amongst the most widely used statistical tests. Chi-square tests always use data based on counts of either people or things. In this chapter we will look at two types of chi-square test: the one-way chi-square test and the chi-square test for association.

Box 16.1 When to use

Use a chi-square test when:

- your variables have been collected using a nominal scale
- you want to see if there is an association between a variable and a particular phenomenon.

Do not convert your data to percentages prior to using the chi-square test.

Chi-square test: one-way

This is probably one of the simplest statistical tests to perform and the basic calculation is as follows:

$$\chi^2 = \Sigma \frac{(O-E)^2}{E}$$

The O stands for observed frequency and the E the expected frequency. The Σ symbol means the sum of. So chi-square is the sum of all the $\frac{(O-E)^2}{E}$ calculations. The important thing to remember about chi-square tests is that they use **frequencies** and if your data are not recorded or can't be converted into frequencies then you can't use chi-square tests. The test is called a one-way test because there is just one variable involved (although this variable may be divided into several categories).

Let's look at an example. Let's say that you are interested in the proportion of people from different ethnic backgrounds who are recruited into nurse training. Obviously ethnicity is nominal-level data and you are looking for an association: is nurse training associated with a particular ethnic group? So you want to use a chi-square test. The hypothesis under test is that there is an association between a particular ethnic group and nurse training. The null hypothesis is, of course, that there is not an association.

Box 16.2 Eye colour and chi-square tests

1. Sample the eye colour of a group of individuals. Test to see if there is a significant association between eye colour and your sample group. Use a chi-square test for homogeneity.
2. Is a chi-square test for homogeneity appropriate? How else could you determine the expected values?

The next step after formulating the hypothesis is to record the number of students of each ethnic group entering nurse education (your population will probably be defined by a geographic area – see Chapter 3). In this case let us say that we are interested in the east London area. These data then become the observations. Below are some hypothetical values. *It is important that you do not convert your data into proportions or percentages.*

TABLE 16.1 The ethnicity of individuals in a cohort entering nurse education

	White (UK and EU)	Afro-Caribbean	Indian sub-continent	Total (from these groups)
Observed	34	62	28	124

For simplicity's sake we have used just three ethnic groups and we look at the ethnicity of a first-year cohort of students training to work with adult patients. These data then become the observations. The expected values that you calculate are dependent on what the theoretical expectations might be. In this example, if there were no association between nurse training and a particular ethnic group it would be reasonable to expect that the ethnic groups should be present in a manner that reflected the local community.

If we take the east London ethnic make-up to be similar to that of the London borough of Hackney we should expect 48 per cent to be white, 33 per cent to be Afro-Caribbean and 19 per cent to be from the Indian sub-continent. We can now calculate the expected frequencies by simply multiplying the total number of students by the proportion for each of the classes (white, Afro-Caribbean and Indian sub-continent). We can thus produce a table that shows both observed and expected frequencies for each category.

TABLE 16.2 Observed and expected frequencies for four ethnic groups in a classroom of students nurses

	White (UK and EU)	Afro-Caribbean	Indian sub-continent	Total (from these groups)
Observed	34	62	28	124
Expected	59.5	41	23.5	124

Having calculated the expected frequencies you can perform the chi-square test as follows:

$$\chi^2 = \Sigma \frac{(O-E)^2}{E} = \frac{(34-59.5)^2}{59.5} + \frac{(62-41)^2}{41} + \frac{(28-23.5)^2}{23.5} =$$

$$\chi^2 = \frac{(-25.5)^2}{59.5} + \frac{(21)^2}{41} + \frac{(4.5)^2}{23.5} =$$

$$\chi^2 = \frac{650.25}{59.5} + \frac{441}{41} + \frac{20.25}{23.5} =$$

$$\chi^2 = 10.9 + 10.7 + 0.86 = 22.46$$

Notice how the values are larger the more the observed value differs from that expected.

Thus $\chi^2 = 22.46$. You must now look up this value in the χ^2 distribution tables, but as with all statistical tests you need to know how many degrees of freedom you have. For the chi-square test for homogeneity, the degrees of freedom are given by the number of categories −1. In this case there are three categories (white, Afro-Caribbean and Indian sub-continent), so there are two degrees of freedom. The χ^2 distribution table, at $P = 0.05$ with two degrees of freedom gives a value of 5.99 (Appendix 3) thus as our value is much larger than this value we can say that there is a significant difference at the $P < 0.05$. In fact our value for χ^2 is greater than the critical value at $P = 0.01$ as well. So we could also say that the difference is significant at $P < 0.01$, and can conclude that there is a significant association between nurse training and ethnic group. There are fewer white (UK and EU) people than expected and more people of Afro-Caribbean origin entering nurse training at this particular site.

Box 16.3 Goodness of fit and chi-square test

You might be asking yourself what is the difference between the test we used for looking at goodness of fit and those described here. The answer is very little. The main difference is that in the goodness of fit tests described earlier the expected values were calculated using a mathematical model not real data. As all mathematical models are hypothetical when we use them to produce expected values, we lose more degrees of freedom than if the expected values are calculated using real data.

A specific type of chi-square exists where the expected categories are all equal. Say, for example, you were looking for an association based on gender, then it would probably be reasonable to suggest that the expected frequencies should be 50 per cent male and 50 per cent female. This type of chi-square where the expected frequencies are equal are known as chi-square tests for homogeneity. The calculations for this test are exactly the same for those described above.

Example from the literature 16.1   Chi-square tests

A relatively simple example of the use of chi-square tests is provided by Shickle et al. (2002). In this study they presented a questionnaire concerning the potential utility of the genetics liaison nurse in running education activities in relation to primary care genetics for primary care health professionals. The questionnaire was very straightforward and they analysed the responses to each question using chi-square tests. Chi-square tests can be used in this way as you can count the type of responses (yes, no, maybe, etc.) to each type of question. In general this approach should not be used for larger questionnaires. The study concluded that at that time the majority of their respondents did not feel there was a need for such an education programme.

Things to look out for

Yates' correction: a correction for limited number of groups

Sometimes when you have just two categories (say you are looking for an association with a particular gender) you will end up having to use just one degree of freedom. In this case a correction must be applied. This correction is called the Yates' correction. The Yates' correction involves a slight alteration to the formula for calculating the chi-square statistic. The new formula is as follows:

$$\chi^2 = \Sigma \frac{(|O - E| - 0.5)^2}{E}$$

You will see that on either side of the symbols for *Observed – Expected*, i.e. O – E of the numerator (the top part of the fraction) there are vertical lines (|), and that this part of the equation is followed by the instruction to subtract 0.5. The vertical bars either side of the O – E tell us to subtract 0.5 from the result of the sum O – E, *ignoring its sign*. Once this process is completed you process the chi-square test as before.

Box 16.4   Practice

Sample the gender of a group of people. Use a chi-square test to see if there is a significant association between a particular gender and the sample.

Take for example the sum below:

$$\frac{(|7-12|-0.5)}{}$$

The answer to this is 4.5. However, the answer to the sum

$$\frac{(7-12-0.5)}{}$$

is -5.5

When using Yates' correction the chi-square values for each calculation use $(|O-E|)-0.5$) as the numerator.

Restrictions on use of the chi-square

If one of your expected frequencies is less than 5 the chi-square test should not be used. Say, for instance in the example used above we had divided the ethnic groups into more precise categories. For example, we could have split the category 'Indian sub-continent' into Bangladeshi, Pakistani, Sikh, Indian Muslim and Indian Hindu. In this case we might find that our categories have expected frequencies of less than 5. As this example demonstrates, one way round this problem is to amalgamate categories (as we did to form 'Indian sub-continent'). The problem with this approach, however, is that the aggregated categories may lose their meaning. It would be very easy to argue that our category 'Indian sub-continent' is so diverse that it is not much use.

If you can't sensibly amalgamate categories, and you have expected frequencies that are less than 5 your only course of action is to use a different test. Options available to you are to use a *G* test or a Fisher's exact test.

Independence

When you use a chi-square-test each datum point must be independent of the others. For example, if you were looking at the use of clinics by different ethnic groups, you would need to exclude return visits by the same individuals. Similarly you need to make sure that the categories are exclusive. There should be no way that an individual could fall into more than one category.

Chi-square test for association: two-way

There are instances when we are interested in more than one nominal scale variable at the same time. For example, we may be interested in whether or not exposure to HIV is associated with particular geographic areas. Here there are two nominal level variables, exposure to HIV and geographic area. In these instances we need to use a two-way chi-square test, often called the chi-square test for association. As with other chi-square tests the basic formula remains the same, i.e.:

$$\chi^2 = \Sigma \frac{(O-E)^2}{E}$$

The difference between the chi-square test for association and those tests described so far is how the expected frequencies are calculated. The method to calculate the expected frequencies is best illustrated through an example.

In the following example we will look at the frequency of cases of multi-drug resistant (MDR) TB across three European countries. In this example we have used genuine data with respect to the proportion of MDR cases (www.eurotb.org) but hypothetical data with respect to the overall number of TB cases. We will look at three countries, Croatia, Czech Republic and Lithuania. We ask the question, is there a significant association between the occurrence of MDR TB and geographic region? The null hypothesis is of course that there is no association and any observed difference is simply caused by sampling error.

Box 16.5

List three pairs of variables that you think it might be interesting to explore if they are associated.

Having established the hypotheses and collected the data the next step is to prepare what is called a contingency table. A contingency table simply sets out the data in a standardized tabular form.

To produce a contingency table the categories from one of the variables are placed in the first row and those from the other variable in the first column. To each first row and column is also added a space for the totals from each row and each column.

TABLE 16.3   A 2 x 3 contingency table showing the incidence of MDR TB in relation to three Eastern European countries

	MDR TB cases	Non-MDR TB cases	Totals
Croatia	13	299	312
Czech Republic	6	184	190
Lithuania	123	170	293
Totals	142	653	795

A Cell → (MDR TB cases, Croatia: 13)

row total → 312

Column total → 142

grand total → 795

This type of table is known as a 2 x 3 contingency table, because we have two column categories and three row categories. If there were just two row categories it would be called a 2 x 2 contingency table.

Box 16.6

Using the following data that relates the experience of childbirth to the type of pain relief used, perform a chi-square test to see if there is an association between the two variables.

Experience	Choice of pain relief		
	Gas+Air	Pethidine	Epidural
1st	66	56	36
2nd +	102	22	12

What problems could there be with this data set with regard to independence?

The next step is to calculate the expected values. Before, when we have used chi-square tests we have already known what the expected values should be. In the examples in the previous section when looking at ethnicity, we used the frequency of the ethnic groups in the community; when looking at sex, we used the approximate global proportions of males and females; and when we used chi-square in goodness of fit test, we used mathematical models. In the case of the chi-square test for association we use the actual data to predict the expected frequencies.

When we calculate the expected frequencies we need to account for the fact that the data is distributed across both the variable country and the variable occurrence of MDR.

We can calculate an expected frequency for each cell by multiplying the total for the cell's row by the total for the cell's column and dividing it by the grand total.

For the highlighted cell in Table 16.3 this calculation would be (312 x 142)/795 = 55.7. Therefore the expected value for this cell is 55.7. This process must be repeated for each cell. We have tabulated the results for our example below.

TABLE 16.4   Expected values for each cell in the contingency table above (Table 16.3)

	MDR TB cases	Non-MDR TB cases
Croatia	55.7	256.3
Czech Republic	33.9	156
Lithuania	52.3	240.7

For each cell we now have to calculate the value give by the formula below:

$$\frac{(O-E)^2}{E}$$

The values for our example are displayed in Table 16.5.

TABLE 16.5   Chi-square calculations for each cell in the contingency Tables 16.3 and 16.4

	MDR TB cases	Non-MDR TB cases
Croatia	32.7	7.1
Czech Republic	23.0	5.0
Lithuania	95.6	20.8

The next step is to add up the all the individual calculations to produce the overall value for chi-square. In this example $\chi^2 = 184$.

Before looking this value up in the chi-square distribution tables you need to work out how many degrees of freedom you have. For chi-square tests of association this is given by $(c - 1)$ x $(r - 1)$, where r refers to the number of row categories and c refers to the number of column categories. In this example this equation gives us $(2 - 1)$ x $(3 - 1) = 2$ degrees of freedom. The critical value from the chi-square table at $P = 0.01$ is 9.21. Our value is much larger than this and therefore we can reject the null hypothesis and say that there is a significant association between geographic area and occurrence of MDR TB. What reasons can you think of that might explain these results?

Box 16.7

1. How many degrees of freedom would you have if the table had been a 2 x 2 contingency table?
2. What do you need to do in such a case? See the first section above.

There are alternatives to using chi-square tests. One often cited by textbooks is the G test. Indeed several statisticians consider that G tests are superior to chi-square tests. However, we have stuck to the traditional approach because you are more likely to come across the chi-square test and few computer packages support G tests. If you would like to read more about the G test Sokal and Rohlf (2012) provides plenty of detail.

Having read this chapter and completed the exercises, you should be familiar with the following ideas and concepts:

- testing for associations;
- calculating expected values;
- testing nominal scale variables;

- Yates' correction;
- restrictions on the use of chi-square test.

1. For the study on the walk-in clinic (Chapter 5) perform an appropriate test to see if the attendance at the clinic is associated with a particular presentation. (a) What happens to the result if you group together those symptoms strongly associated with sexually transmitted diseases? (b) What explanations do you think there are for this relationship? (c) Is choice of contraceptive related to ethnicity? (d) What explanations do you think there are for this association?
2. Is there an association between ethnic group and sex with respect to attendance at the clinic? What explanations do you think there are for this difference?
3. Sample the eye colour of a group of individuals. Test to see if there is a significant association between eye colour and your sample group. Use a chi-square test for homogeneity. Is a chi-square test for homogeneity appropriate? How else could you determine the expected values?

17

Tests for association: correlation and regression

Areas of learning covered in this chapter

- How do I see if two variables show a linear relationship?
- What are correlation and regression?
- How are regression and correlation used? How are they related? And how can they be used to make predictions?
- What types of restrictions are there on the use of regression analysis?

In the previous chapter we looked at tests for association for variables measured on the nominal scale, e.g. chi-square. In this chapter we look at the test most frequently used to test for association for variables that are measured on the interval and ordinal scales. This means that the way the calculations are made is quite different from the way we calculated nominal data and how we tested for associations between variables.

The main test for association we will look at is called Pearson's correlation. In principle Pearson's correlation should be used with interval scale data (parametric). Pearson's correlation can also be used for data gathered on the ordinal scale (non-parametric) when the sample size is greater than thirty. When using data gathered on the ordinal scale, if the sample size is less than thirty the Spearman's rank correlation should be used (Chapter 15). Pearson's correlation is used to determine the extent to which a change in one variable tends to be associated with a change in another. The correlation techniques we demonstrate will seek to test for linear correlation, that is whether the variables are associated along a straight line continuum. Where one variable is associated with another in this way they are said to be correlated.

It is perfectly possible to have non-linear correlations and there are statistical procedures to test for them. They are, however, beyond the scope of this book. If you are interested in following this up see Bates and Watts (1988).

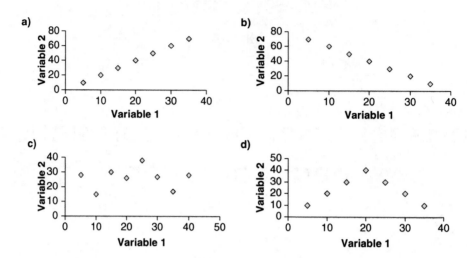

FIGURE 17.1   Different forms of correlation: (a) positive linear correlation; (b) negative linear
correlation; (c) no correlation; (d) canonical correlation. Note that there are many
different types of non-linear correlation

A correlation can be either positive or negative. A positive correlation is where as the cases of one variable increase so do those in the other. For example, there is a correlation between age and occurrence of breast cancer. As age *increases* so the incidence of breast cancer increases.

Sometimes we may find a decrease in one variable as another variable increases. For example, there is an association between increasing wealth and decreasing incidence of mental health problems. This is known as a negative correlation.

Regression in some respects is as much a descriptive statistic as it is an inferential one. Regression is a technique whereby the line that best fits the points on the graph is determined. It is only appropriate to perform a regression analysis if you want to predict the value of one variable from another or you think that the parameters of the line have a significant bearing on your study.

Box 17.1   Correlations (I)

Suggest:

- three positive correlations between two variables;
- three negative correlation between two variables;
- one non-linear regression.

Correlation

When we perform a correlation we not only ask if there is a correlation but we also want to know how strong the relationship is. The correlation test asks how strong the relationship is and whether the correlation is greater than could be expected by chance. The correlations shown in Figures 17.1a and b are perfect correlations. By this we mean that *all* the variation in variable 2 can be explained by the variation in variable 1. If the points were much more scattered the correlation would be weaker, until the scatter is such that there is no relationship. This is the case in Figure 17.1c. Scatter can be caused by error or by the fact that there are other factors which influence the variation in a particular variable. If we take breast cancer, for example, we know that there are other factors besides age which can influence whether or not an individual suffers from breast cancer, thus it is unlikely that if we correlated age with breast cancer we would get a perfect correlation. Note that in correlation for every point plotted we have a value from each variable. The values are paired.

Box 17.2 Correlations (II)

Try to find three articles where the idea of correlation is discussed.
   Reflect on these articles and consider how the correlation is used by the authors and whether their conclusions are justified

---

The statistic that we calculate to determine the strength of a correlation is called the Pearson's correlation coefficient. It is also known as the product moment correlation. It has the symbol r. To perform the Pearson's correlation you must know that both variables approximate to (are not significantly different from) the normal distribution (see Chapter 14). In many studies where Pearson's correlation is used the authors do not check for normality.

How to calculate the Pearson's correlation coefficient (r)

First of all you need some data. In general you want a sample with at least thirty pairs of samples. In this example we will use just ten, but this is just for simplicity.

Abdo Sadu is a public health officer specializing in respiratory problems and is conducting some research investigating various aspects of lung function and pollution levels. As part of his study he is seeking to establish if there is a relationship between levels of atmospheric sulphur dioxide levels SO_2 and peak flow. Sulphur dioxide is an atmospheric pollutant associated with the burning of oil and coal. Peak flow is the maximum instantaneous rate that an individual can expel air out of his lungs.

The first step, as we suggest when dealing with most aspects of statistics, is to plot out the data. The plot suggests that there is an association (relationship). However, could it just be due to chance, i.e. error in the sampling process?

The next step would be to test for normality with respect to both the variables, which we discussed in Chapter 14. For the purposes of saving space we will omit this stage.

Now we can get on with calculating r. The procedure is similar to that for the ANOVA test (Chapter 13) in that it involves using the sums of squares. We need to do this for both variables.

TABLE 17.1 Mean pollution levels across ten US cities and the mean peak flow recorded in those cities from women aged twenty-five

Pollution level (µg/m³) in ten US cities	Peak flow (mls/sec) – average for females aged twenty-five
47	40
9	55
14	50
11	52
23	42
17	44
56	40
110	38
30	44
23	42

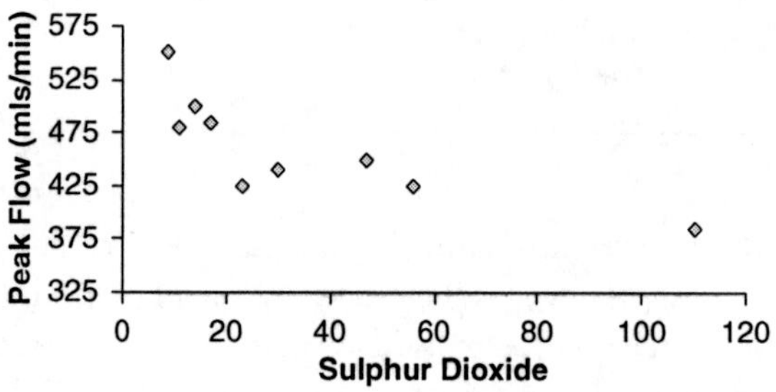

FIGURE 17.2 Relationship between peak flow and pollution levels

When we are doing the calculation we will refer to the variables by the letters x and y. Traditionally x is the variable that we plot on the horizontal axis and y is the variable we plot on the vertical axis. It is normal to plot the variable on the x-axis that you think gives rise to the effect. This variable is sometimes called the independent variable. In correlation, however, it doesn't matter which variable you select to be the x-axis. In regression it does!

The calculation you need to perform is to calculate the sums of squares of the cases of the x variable, then the y variable. You then need to calculate the result of multiplying each pair of x and y together. We recommend using a table as set out in Table 17.2.

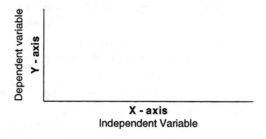

FIGURE 17.3 Axes of the independent and dependent variables

TABLE 17.2   Calculation table for Pearson's correlation coefficient

	Pollution level (μg/m³)	Peak flow (mls/sec)	x^2	y^2	xy (x and y multiplied together)
Case pair 1	47	40	2209	1600	1880
Case pair 2	9	55	81	3025	495
Case pair 3	14	50	196	2500	700
Case pair 4	11	52	121	2704	572
Case pair 5	23	42	529	1764	966
Case pair 6	17	44	289	1936	748
Case pair 7	56	40	3136	1600	2240
Case pair 8	110	38	12100	1444	4180
Case pair 9	30	44	900	1936	1320
Case pair 10	23	42	529	1764	966
Totals (Σ)	340 (Σx)	447(Σy)	20090 (Σx²)	20273 (Σy²)	14067 (Σxy)

As with most statistics, the advantages of using a computer soon become apparent. We used Microsoft Excel to perform the calculations shown in Table 17.2. Using a spreadsheet helps to reduce the number of errors that are made.

Box 17.3

Take samples from a group of people of index and little finger length. Are these measurements significantly correlated?

The next step is to calculate the sum of the *xs* squared ((Σx)²) and the sum of the *ys* squared ((Σy)²). These values are 115600 (340²) and 199809 (447²) respectively.

The next step is to calculate the statistic *r*, the correlation coefficient. This is calculated according to the formula below. Like most statistical formulas it looks more frightening than it is. If you can add up, divide, subtract and multiply then you can do it.

$$r = \frac{n \times \sum xy - \left(\sum x \times \sum y \right)}{\sqrt{\left[n \times \sum x^2 - \left(\sum x \right)^2 \right]\left[n \times \sum y^2 - \left(\sum y \right)^2 \right]}}$$

Feeding our values into the equation we have:

$$r = \frac{10 \times 14067 - (340 \times 447)}{\sqrt{\left[10 \times 20090 - (115600) \right]\left[10 \times 20273 - (199809) \right]}}$$

After performing the multiplications inside brackets:

$$r = \frac{14670 - (151980)}{\sqrt{[200900 - (115600)][202730 - (199809)]}}$$

After performing the subtractions (remember to do the subtractions in brackets first):

$$r = \frac{-11310}{\sqrt{[85300][2921]}}$$

Now you can perform the final multiplication to give:

$$r = \frac{-11310}{\sqrt{249161300}}$$

Next square root the denominator:

$$r = \frac{-11310}{15784.8}$$

And finally calculate r:

$$r = 0.71$$

The significance of r, i.e. is there a statistically significant correlation, just like any other statistic, can be read from tables that show the critical values for of r (see Appendix 3). In a correlation the number of degrees of freedom are given by the sample size minus the number of variables. There are two variables in this case so we therefore have eight degrees of freedom. So looking up an r of -0.71 with eight degrees of freedom we see that the relationship is significant at the $P < 0.05$, but not at the $P < 0.01$ level. The correlation is thus significant but not very strong. It should be noted, however, that this test was a two-tailed test (i.e. we did not predict whether the relationship would be positive or negative and would be a more significant relationship if the test was one-tailed). Notice also that the relationship is negative, thus as x gets bigger y gets smaller.

Some studies report a t value as well as the r value. We will not outline the procedure here except to say that the t value calculated is derived from r and most computer packages will produce both.

The coefficient of determination

One very simple add-on to a correlation test is to produce what is called the coefficient of determination. This is simply the regression coefficient squared. Notice when you do this the coefficient of determination (r^2) is always smaller than r (except when $r = 1$). What does this new statistic tell us? It tells us the percentage of the variation in one variable that is explained by the other. In the study described above the coefficient of determination is 0.50. This suggests that for our sample 50 per cent of the variation in peak flow can be attributed to the levels of sulphur dioxide in the atmosphere.

Box 17.4 Limitations

1. You can't tell that a relationship is 'cause and effect' just because you have a correlation.
2. Measurements must be interval or ratio scales.
3. Samples must have been taken randomly and normally distributed.
4. You can't use time as a variable on the x-axis.
5. Make sure you plot your data before you do a correlation. The relationship should be linear, although you can transform some types of relationship (see below).

Use correlation when you have samples in excess of thirty. If you have fewer cases use the Spearman's rank correlation.

Example from the literature 17.1 Pearson correlation

Correlation techniques are quite commonly used in exploratory research, sometimes involving large sets of data. Collison et al. (2007) investigated the association between wealth inequalities and various measures of population health. For instance, they explored the relationship between the level of inequality and infant mortality. Both these variables seem to produce data that approximates to the normal distribution and are therefore suitable for Pearson correlation. This study is particularly interesting because they remove data points that they thought could be having a strong influence on the overall patterns they were observing and then reanalysed their data. This is good practice and is an important step in trying to establish the underlying causes behind an observed association. This paper can be accessed at: http://intl-jpubhealth.oxfordjournals.org/content/29/2/114.full.

Regression

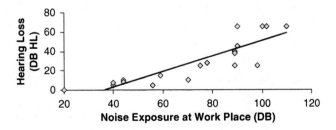

FIGURE 17.4   Noise exposure and hearing loss

Regression analysis is a technique used to determine the best position to put a line through a group of points on a scatter graph. You will want to know this if you want to show a relationship graphically or express it mathematically. Once a relationship is expressed in this way you can use the relationship to make predictions. What is more you can use the regression analysis to help express the degree of confidence that you have in a prediction. You may also want to know where a line should be placed if you are interested in having a fundamental understanding of the nature of the relationship between the variables that are being studies. As with correlation, to perform a regression analysis you need to have measures of two different variables from the same sampling unit. Each single measure of one variable has a pair derived from the other measured variable.

Regression analysis can be used on many types of relationship but here we will confine ourselves to linear regression.

Box 17.5 Relationships

Think of three relationships between variables that are commonly used in the field of health.

How were these relationships determined?

Investigate one of these relationships and explore the nature of the sampling regime.

As with most analyses in statistics the calculations look much harder than they are, and basic mathematical skills will be sufficient but a computer helps even more.

The line

The line through the points is really a slope. It could be a flat slope or a very steep slope. What regression analysis essentially tries to do is to find a slope where each datum point has an equal influence over where the slope should be. This line is known as the 'line of best fit'. Regression analysis can also tell us other useful parameters such as how accurate a prediction would be based on the line of best fit.

What is a slope?

A slope is really a mathematical description of the relationship between two variables. You may have heard of the term gradient when talking about steep hills. Gradient and slope mean the same thing. In talking about a hill the gradient or slope is a unit of distance along the vertical divided by the amount of distance one would need to travel to descend or climb that distance.

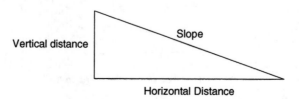

FIGURE 17.5 Slope

$$Slope = \frac{Vertical\ distance}{Horizontal\ distance}$$

In the example above if you moved 30 m along the horizontal in order to descend 5 m the slope would be:

$$Slope = \frac{5}{30}$$

which would equal 0.167.

The point about the slope is that it allows you to predict the distance you need to travel in order to descend a certain amount. So if you wanted to go down 110.5 metres, we could predict the distance you need to travel along the horizontal.

We do this by rearranging the equation

$$Slope = \frac{Vertical\ distance}{Horizontal\ distance} \quad to \quad Horizontal\ distance = \frac{Vertical\ distance}{Slope}$$

so in this case where we want to descend 110.5 metres and the slope is 0.167 then we would need to travel 661.7 metres along the horizontal. We could also predict the amount of the descent given a known distance of travel along the horizontal. To do this the equation would be rearranged to

$$Vertical\ distance = Horizontal\ distance \times Slope$$

When we carry out regression analysis we are normally interested in being able to predict a value on the vertical axis for a given value on the horizontal axis. You will recall that in graphs we call the vertical axis the y-axis and the horizontal axis the x-axis. Using the letters y and x to mean the vertical (y) and horizontal (x) respectively. Our equation for predicting a value of x from a value of y becomes:

$Y = Slope.x$

($y = x$ multiplied by the slope)

The equations above tell us the amount we need to move along one axis in relation to the amount we need to move along another. They will only actually predict the exact value of say y for a given value of x in one circumstance, and that is where the start point is zero (i.e. the data pass through what is called the origin of the graph).

Unfortunately, most data we deal with does not pass through the origin, so we must adjust our equation accordingly. Think of a relationship between, for example, exercise level (running speed) and oxygen consumption. We would expect oxygen consumption to rise with exercise level (as energy demand increases), but even at a zero level of exercise we would still expect

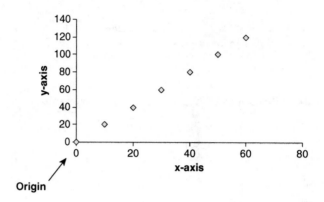

FIGURE 17.6 The origin of a graph

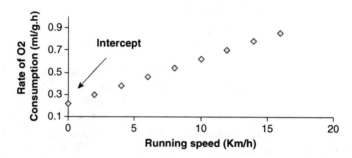

FIGURE 17.7 The intercept of a graph

a person to be using oxygen! The relationship between exercise level and oxygen consumption would therefore not pass through the origin. If we tried to predict oxygen consumption from exercise level using the equation described above it would not work. It wouldn't work because our y-axis (oxygen consumption) would not pass through zero. The point at which the slope would cross the y axis is known as the intercept.

To be able to predict a value for oxygen consumption from running speed one would need to start not at zero but at the intercept. Our equation above that related x and y via the slope needs to include the intercept. The new equation is:

$y = \text{intercept} + \text{slope}.x$

It is normal in statistics to refer to the slope by the letter b and the intercept by the letter a. Thus our equation becomes $y = a + bx$.

Regression analysis is about finding the optimum values for both the slope (b) and the intercept (a).

Linear regression comes in two forms, model 1 and model 2 regression. Model 1 is the option most researchers use mainly because it is available on most computer packages. It is not always the correct choice. We will discuss model 1 regression with examples and then go on to outline model 2.

> # Box 17.6 Investigating slopes
>
> For the relationship you explored in Box 17.5, find the slope (by hand not by statistics) and express the relationship between the variables in terms of the equation of a straight line. Try to determine the slope of a flight of stairs, or the slope of a ruler on your desk.

The analysis (model 1)

Kavita Patel is a dietician working with patients suffering from obesity. She is interested in the weight loss that is associated with calorie-restricted diets. Kavita establishes a study in which 100 obese people are allocated to each of ten different diet groups. Kavita assumes that a reduced calorie diet regime will lead to weight loss but she wants to know how much to reduce a diet by to produce a certain weight loss.

Each diet is essentially the same but the amount of calories available in each varies, between 1000 and 2000 kcals. All Kavita's participants are male and are in the age range of forty-five to fifty. All have been referred to Kavita by their doctors and have agreed to take part in the study. Kavita weighed her participants at the beginning of the study and then eight weeks into the diet.

The main function with a regression analysis is to determine the position of the parameters *a* (intercept) and *b* (slope). However, we would also be interested in whether or not the relationship in question is statistically significant, i.e. is the slope significantly different from 0. Therefore, Kavita's null hypothesis is that there is no significant linear relationship between calorific content of a diet regime and weight loss.

The type of regression analysis that we will describe is called the least squares method, and what this techniques does is to place a line (mathematically) through points on a scattergram such that the sum of the distance (vertical) between all the points and the line is minimum. The significance of this approach is that it attempts to minimize the error on the *y*-axis and assumes that the *x*-axis values are measured without error. Unlike correlation however the data on the *x*-axis does not need to be normally distributed.

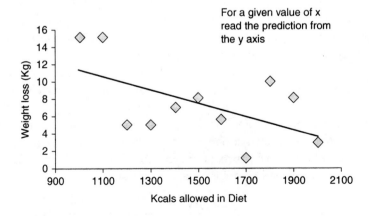

FIGURE 17.8 Reading a prediction from a regression equation

TABLE 17.3 Values for weight loss associated with a particular level of calorie intake restricted diet

Diet	Weight loss (kg)
1000	15
1100	15
1200	5
1300	5
1400	7
1500	8
1600	5.5
1700	1
1800	10
1900	8
2000	3

Table 17.3 shows the data from Kavita's study. The diet is the independent variable and the weight loss the dependent variable, the assumption being that the weight loss is associated with a particular diet and that the amount of weight loss is dependent on the diet. In regression analysis the x axis should always be that which is thought to be the independent variable. In some cases there may not be an independent variable, in which case the y variable should be the one that you want to make predictions of from a given value of x.

The first step in any regression analysis should be to plot the data. In this way you can get a 'feel' for the data and a preliminary idea of what the statistics might show. You can also check for outliers, which are data points which do not seem to fit the prevailing trend. Care does need to be taken when deciding if a point is an outlier when using small data sets. In a small data set, one could argue that the overall trend cannot be seen and therefore it is inappropriate to call any point an outlier.

Having looked at the data you need to decide if a linear relationship is reasonable. Do consider other relationships between variables like those described at the start of this chapter. If you decide that linear regression is the best option you can then press on with the calculations to calculate a least squares regression and find values for the slope and the intercept.

The calculation of a least squares regression is quite similar to that for correlation, so you need to find the same parameters (sums of squares for x and y) as you did for correlation. Table 17.4 shows the production of these parameters for Kavita's data.

You also need to find the mean of all the x and the y values, and also the square of the sum of the x values $(\Sigma x)^2$. We calculated all the values used using an Excel spreadsheet. If you don't have access to a statistical package but do have access to a computer, using a spreadsheet speeds up calculations and reduces errors. For Kavita's data $\bar{x} = 1500$ $\bar{y} = 7.5$ and $(\Sigma x)^2 = 272{,}250{,}000$.

Having calculated the parameters as normal the next step is to put those parameters into the equations that will enable the final statistics to be produced. The first step is to calculate the value of the slope. As we said previously, in statistics this has the symbol b.

$$b = \frac{n \times \Sigma xy - \Sigma x \times \Sigma y}{n \times \Sigma x^2 - (\Sigma x)^2}$$

TABLE 17.4 Calculation table for least squares regression

	Diet (kcal) (x)	Weight loss (kg) (y)	x^2	y^2	xy (x and y multiplied together)
Case pair 1	1000	15	1000000	225	15000
Case pair 2	1100	15	1210000	225	16500
Case pair 3	1200	5	1440000	25	6000
Case pair 4	1300	5	1690000	25	6500
Case pair 5	1400	7	1960000	49	9800
Case pair 6	1500	8	2250000	64	12000
Case pair 7	1600	5.5	2560000	30.25	8800
Case pair 8	1700	1	2890000	1	1700
Case pair 9	1800	10	3240000	100	18000
Case pair 10	1900	8	3610000	64	15200
Case pair 11	2000	3	4000000	9	6000
Totals (Σ)	16500 (Σx)	82.5 (Σy)	25850000 (Σx^2)	817.25 (Σy^2)	115500 (Σxy)

Using the values from Kavita's study this gives us

$$b = \frac{(11 \times 115500) - (16500 \times 82.5)}{(11 \times 25850000) - (272250000)} = \frac{(1270500) - (1361250)}{(284350000) - (272250000)}$$

which equals

$$b = \frac{-90750}{12100000}$$

therefore

$$b = -0.0075$$

The minus indicates that the slope is negative, i.e. as we move up the x-axis the slope goes down.

Having calculated b it is now possible to calculate a, the intercept, by solving the equation for a straight line. If you remember the equation is $y = a + bx$, where b and a are the slope and intercept respectively. If we take the mean y values, the mean of the x values and the value for b we have calculated and put them into the equation we have:

$$7.5 = a + -0.0075 \times 1500$$

We thus have an equation where the only parameter we don't know is a. With a little rearrangement we can get to:

$$a = y - bx$$

Substituting our values produces:

$$a = 7.5 - -0.0075 \times 1500$$

which equals:

$$a = 7.5 + 11.25$$

and thus $a = 18.75$

Our final equation for Kavita's data is thus

$$y = 18.75 - 0.0075x$$

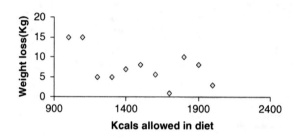

FIGURE 17.9   The relationship between kcals in diet and weight loss

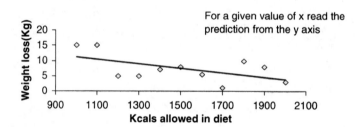

FIGURE 17.10   Reading a prediction from a regression equation

If you want to make a prediction using the line take a value of x, in the case of Kavita's work, a diet of a certain calorific content, and then use the equation make a prediction. So for a value of x of 1200, Kavita's equation predicts a weight loss of 9.75 kg.

You could also make a prediction by drawing the line on the original graph. To do this make a prediction for a value of x at both extremes of the range of the x values. Plot the prediction on the graph and join the two points together with a straight line. You can then read from the straight line a prediction for any given value of x. But how good is that estimate?

Quality of a prediction

It is important to remember that a regression line is a statistic. Not only that but normally it is a statistic based on a sample, in Kavita's case a sample of obese individuals. When we produce a regression line from a sample, just like when we produce a mean from a sample, it is an estimate of where the line would lie for the population as a whole. This means that a prediction will carry error. In fact any prediction will carry with it two types of error: the error caused by the fact that we are using a sample and the error caused by the scatter of points around the line.

The 95 per cent confidence limits (Chapter 11) for an individual prediction are given by the equation below:

$$95 \text{ per cent confidence limit (CL }_{95\%}) = y' \pm t \times s_r \sqrt{1 + \frac{1}{n} + \frac{(x' - \bar{x})^2}{\Sigma x^2 - \frac{(\Sigma x)^2}{n}}}$$

You will have met all the symbols before except for x', y' and s_r. The symbol x' tells us that we are referring to a single value of x and the y' a single value of y. It is of course the y value predicted by the value of x. The s_r in the equation is the standard error of the regression line and, just like the standard error of the mean discussed in earlier chapters, it is a measure of how close the estimated value for the slope is to that of the true population. You may remember that s normally denotes some sort of variance and indeed s_r is derived from the residual variance s_r^2. The value of t used is that from the statistical tables for the distribution of t (see Appendix 3) for the appropriate degrees of freedom. In regression analysis with two variables this is given by $n - 2$.

Box 17.7 Regression

From the data that you collected for the exercise in Box 17.3 calculate a regression line, using the index figure as the x-axis.

Predict the length of an individual's little finger whose index finger is 7 cm.

How accurate is your prediction?

The residual variance s_r^2 is calculated using the equations below:

$$s_r^2 = \frac{1}{n-2} \left(\Sigma y^2 - \frac{(\Sigma y)^2}{n} - \frac{\left(\Sigma xy - \frac{\Sigma x \Sigma y}{n} \right)^2}{\Sigma x^2 - \frac{(\Sigma x)^2}{n}} \right)$$

As with most statistical equations there is nothing more than the standard mathematical functions to do here, but it is quite complex and working by hand you need to take it one step at a time and be patient. Below we calculate s_r^2 for Kavita's data. Fortunately, the only new parameter we need to calculate is $\left(\Sigma y\right)^2$. The others can come from Table 17.4. We will show some, but to save space, not all the steps.

$$s_r^2 = \frac{1}{9} \times \left(817.25 - \frac{6806.25}{11} - \frac{\left(115500 - \frac{16500 \times 82.5}{11} \right)^2}{25850000 - \frac{272250000}{11}} \right)$$

$$s_r^2 = \frac{1}{9} \times \left(817.25 - 618.75 - \frac{\left(115500 - 123750 \right)^2}{1100000} \right)$$

$$s_r^2 = \frac{1}{9} \times \left(817.25 - 618.75 - 61.875 \right) = s_r^2 = 0.111 \times 136.25$$

$$s_r^2 = 15.123$$

Thus $s_r = \sqrt{15.123} = 3.88$

This value is the standard error of the slope. In other words, we are saying that we are about 66 per cent confident that the position of the slope of the population is anywhere in the range of -0.0075 ± 3.88.

To calculate the confidence limits for a particular estimate we must plug the value we have for the standard error of the slope into equation x (below) which was outlined above:

95 per cent confidence limit of an estimate $(CL_{95\%}) = y' \pm t \times s_r \sqrt{1 + \frac{1}{11} + \frac{(x' - \bar{x})^2}{\Sigma x^2 - \frac{(\Sigma x)^2}{n}}}$

In the example below Kavita is interested in a prediction based on an x value of 1200. From the equation for her regression line this gives her a predicted y value of 9.75.

$$CL_{95\%} = 9.75 \pm t \times 3.88 \sqrt{1 + \frac{1}{11} + \frac{(1200 - 1500)^2}{25850000 - \frac{272250000}{11}}}$$

$$CL_{95\%} = 9.75 \pm t \times 3.88 \sqrt{1 + 0.091 + \frac{90000}{1100000}}$$

$$CL_{95\%} = 9.75 \pm t \times 3.88 \sqrt{1.172}$$

$$CL_{95\%} = 9.75 \pm t \times 3.88 \times 1.08$$

t at $P = 0.05$ (95 per cent confidence) $= 2.306$

thus the 95 per cent CL for a prediction based on 1200 calories is

9.75kg $\pm$ 9.67

Is the relationship between the variables significant?

If you were Kavita you might now be thinking that this is a fairly poor prediction, and you would probably check to see if the regression between the two variables was actually significant. We check this by calculating a t value for the slope. The equation for this is as follows:

$$t = b \times \sqrt{\frac{\sum x^2 - \frac{(\sum x)^2}{n}}{S_r^2}}$$

The values from Kavita's study are as follows:

$$t = -0.0075 \times \sqrt{\frac{25850000 - \frac{272250000}{11}}{15.123}} = t = -0.0075 \times \sqrt{\frac{25850000 - \frac{272250000}{11}}{15.123}}$$

$$t = -0.0075 \times \sqrt{72736.89} = -.0075 \times 269.69$$

$$t = -2.022$$

This value can now be looked up in the t distribution tables (ignore the minus sign) The critical value at $P = 0.05$ and eight degrees of freedom is 2.262. As such the calculated value of t is less than the critical value and we can say that the slope of the relationship between the two variables does not significantly differ from zero, and therefore diet type (calorific content) is not a good predictor of weight loss.

Box 17.8 Regression

From the data that you collected for the exercise in Box 17.3 that you have calculated a regression line for determine if the variables are significantly correlated.

You are probably thinking that we have produced a lot of calculations to reach the conclusion that the variables are not significant. However, we wanted to go through the process of forming an estimation for the parameters of the slope first in order to emphasize that the focus of bivariate (two variables) linear regression analysis should be the slope rather than if there is a relationship. It would be wise, however, if working without a statistics package, if you have doubts, to test if there is a relationship before proceeding with a determination of the slope. In practice, when asked to perform a regression analysis, most computer packages will produce all the required statistics, including regression coefficients and coefficients of determination.

As well as producing error estimates for the slope it is also possible to do this for the intercept term b. For the sake of economy we will not discuss these here, but details can be found in Sokal and Rohlf (2012). Most statistical packages will produce error statistics for the intercept alongside the other regression statistics.

Box 17.9 Restrictions on the use of least squares regression

1. Use linear regression only when you believe that the relationship between the variables (after transforming if necessary) conforms to a linear type model.
2. The data should be measured on the interval or ratio scales.
3. The level of error in the y-axis should be constant across the range of y-values, i.e. the level of scatter should be constant either side of the line across the whole distance of the line. If it isn't don't use least squares regression analysis; try Spearman's rank instead.
4. Regression makes no assumptions about normality on the x-axis, and so can be used in situations where time forms the x-axis.
5. When quoting the statistics for a regression analysis, quote the equation for the slope. If it is significant and at what level, give a P value and the sample size. Oddly, the correlation coefficient (r) has no meaning in regression analysis but is often quoted. If quoting a prediction from a regression equation the error of estimation should always be quoted.

Model 2 regression

When you are regressing two variables together, whether to use type 2 regression is a consideration only when you are interested in the functional significance of the slope. This could be the case if you wanted to understand why a certain variable, say metabolic rate, increases with increasing body mass. Here you want to go beyond description and prediction and toward understanding. The first type of regression we described is perfectly adequate in most situations. In a few cases, however, type 2 regression is required.

Box 17.10 Model 2 regression

Using the data from the two previous boxes decide which regression model should best be used to determine the functional significance of the regression line.

The most common situation it is required in is where both the x and the y variables are measured randomly and the level of error in the measurement of both is similar. In type 1 regression the position of the line takes into account sampling error on the x-axis only, and thus if both axis are measured with similar levels of error, the line will not be positioned correctly.

You will recall that in Kavita's data set she assigned diets to individuals and thus the x-axis is not a randomly measured variable. In addition, because she determined the kcals within the diet the level of sample error on the x-axis is low (although measurement error could be high is the participants didn't adhere to their diets). Kavita was also more concerned with making predictions than the functional relationship between the variables. Therefore, for Kavita, type 1 regression is appropriate. An example where you would use model 2 regression is where you were interested in the size of a particular type of cancerous growth and exposure to radiation. Here both axes are likely to be randomly sampled and be normally distributed.

Unfortunately most computer programs do not easily enable the computation of type 2 regression, and therefore model 1 regression analysis is sometimes used inappropriately. A quick 'rough and ready' method to determine the slope in situations where a model 2 regression is required is to divide the slope by r, the correlation coefficient. Alternative and more sophisticated methods do exist, for example Bartlett's three-group method, Kendall's robust line fit method and major axis regression (Kendall's robust line fit method is a non-parametric method).

Not linear

It is important to remember that linear regression is an approach that assumes your data conforms to a linear model (i.e. falls approximately along a straight line). This is why it is important to plot your data before you do anything else.

In many cases your data will not be linear (e.g. bacterial growth over time) and, as such, in the first instance, linear regression is not appropriate. Computer statistics packages do often have facilities for performing what is known as 'non-linear regression'. However, the use of these techniques and their interpretation is rather complex. In addition if you do not have access to such packages then an alternative strategy is required.

Fortunately, for many types of non-linear relationship between variables it is possible to transform the data so that the relationship between the variables takes on a linear form. Shown below is the relationship between metabolic rate and body weight for adult males. Clearly for these, data linear regression would not be appropriate unless we transform the data such that they become linear.

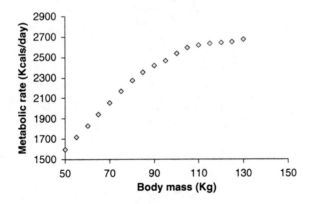

FIGURE 17.9 The relationship between body mass and metabolic rate

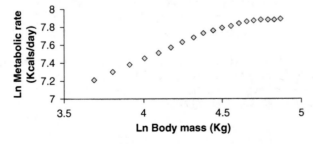

FIGURE 17.10 The relationship between body mass and metabolic rate

To straighten this type of curve (often called asymptotic) we can take the natural logarithm of both the *x* and the *y*-axes. The resulting curve is shown in Figure 17.10.

The line is not completely straight but it is suitable for regression analysis based on a linear model. If you perform such an analysis the resulting line will have the formula:

Ln Metabolic rate = $a + b$ x Ln Body mass.

Other common forms of transformation include logging just one of the axes, the reciprocal transformation (take the reciprocal of the *y*-axis) and the probit transformation. (For information on these see Sokal and Rohlf 2012.)

Multiple regression

Sometimes we are interested in phenomena that may be affected by and correlated with a variety of different variables. For example, in thinking of a person's chance of getting heart disease, we know there are a range of important independent variables such as smoking, amount of exercise taken and obesity that are correlated with the risk of suffering from a myocardial infarction. The technique we need to use if we want to consider the influence of a variety of independent variables on a dependent variable is called multiple regression. Multiple regression is a common technique but beyond the scope of this book. If you wish to investigate further try Allison (1999).

Having read this chapter and completed the exercises, you should be familiar with the following ideas and concepts:

- testing for associations;
- using correlation;
- using least squares linear regression;
- the coefficient of determination;
- the correlation coefficient;
- the difference between correlation and regression;
- making predictions using least squares regression;
- determining the accuracy of predictions made using least squares;
- model 2 regression;
- transforming non-linear relationships.

1. For the study on Symphadiol presented in Chapter 5 perform an appropriate test to see if the weight loss of the participant significantly correlates with the height of the participant. (a) Plot the relationship. (b) What explanations do you think there are for this relationship? (c) Is the relationship a strong one? (d) Predict the weight of an individual who is 170 cm tall. (e) What do you think gives rise to the variations around the slope? (f) What is the standard error of the slope you have calculated?

2. Identify three studies from the literature in which least squares regression is used. For each study: (a) note the size of the sample; (b) indicate if the restrictions on least squares regression have been adhered to; (c) if the test selection was inappropriate, discuss how you believe this could change the conclusions.

18

How big a sample: power analysis

Areas of learning covered in this chapter

- Why determining sample size is important.
- What is statistical power?
- How to estimate an appropriate sample size to use when predicting population means.
- How to estimate sample sizes when performing statistical tests.
- What is effect size and why is it important to consider?

The statistical tests that we have described in this book rely on the sample used being drawn randomly from the population(s) under study. The power of the test, that is the ability to detect a statistical difference or association if one is present, relies largely on three factors: the type of statistical test, the size of the sample taken and the extent of the variation within the variable under investigation (see Chapter 3).

It is not always easy to know at the outset of a study quite how large a sample size is needed and it is very disappointing when looking at the result of a study to find that, although the data show a difference, it is not statistically significant, and to be left thinking, 'If only I had taken a larger sample'. Conversely if you take too many samples, you will be using participants and resources unnecessarily which could be considered ethically dubious.

Power is lost when the sample size does not adequately reflect the population. Samples are taken of the population, because normally the resources are not available to collect data from the entire population. For a statistical test to have power, the sample must be representative of the population (Figure 18.1). Power analysis can be used, with respect to the variable of interest, to predict the size of sample required and the extent to which a certain sample size will be representative of the population as a whole.

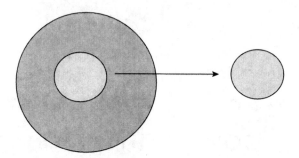

FIGURE 18.1   Diagrammatic representation of a sample (small circle) being drawn from a population (large circle). We normally sample from a population as often we do not have the resources to work on the whole population. For most, but not all, quantitative work the sample should be drawn randomly from the population

The main difficulty with **power analysis** is that it requires prior information with regard to two factors: first, you need to know the likely level variation in the variable of interest; and second, you must have some idea of the minimum size of the difference that you are interested in detecting.

The first factor (variability) is simply an estimate of the likely standard deviation. This estimate can be obtained either from previous published studies of the variable of interest or by conducting a small pilot study. Deciding on a minimum size of the difference is more difficult; sometimes in a study you may just be looking for any significant difference, while at other times you may be guided more by what is likely to be significant in terms of health practice (see discussion in Chapter 9). In essence however, this question is asking how large a margin of error you are prepared to tolerate.

To explore power analysis further, we will first look at predicting a sample size, when we are simply trying to predict the arithmetic mean of a population from a sample, and then go on to look at how sample size can be determined when using statistical tests for examining hypotheses.

Basic power analysis: sample size prediction when predicting a population mean from a sample

The equation for a simple power analysis to determine the sample size for estimating a population mean is relatively straightforward although it introduces some terms that you may not initially be familiar with: chiefly the term B, which we have not used in this text so far. B stands for boundary. The B is set at your reasonable margin of error. The other term used, which we have discussed little thus far, is alpha (α). Alpha is simply the probability of committing a type I error. A type I error is the rejection of a null hypothesis when it is in fact true. In statistical testing when we set the acceptance level at $P = 0.05$, we are also effectively setting the acceptable alpha level, which is therefore 0.05. The equation for this basic sample size analysis is:

$$\left(z_{\alpha/2} \frac{\sigma}{B} \right)^2 < n$$

The first part of the equation tells us that we need to select a z value for the level of alpha that we require; obviously the higher the alpha, the higher the sample size needed. The z value chosen should reflect the confidence limit (see Chapter 11) that you will use eventually to express the accuracy of the sample mean relative to the population mean.

To find the z value, all you need to do is to divide the chosen alpha by two, and then locate this number in the table for the z distribution (Table 11.1), read the relevant column heading and the row heading to give the z value. In the case of a desired alpha of 0.05 (giving a confidence limit of 95 per cent) the value is 1.96.

Having obtained the appropriate z value, the next step is to find an estimate for sigma (σ). Sigma is the standard deviation for the population. Of course, if you had this value then you probably would not need to do a power test as you would not need to do any sampling. In reality therefore the value used is an estimate, which is normally based on either a prior study of the same variable, or a pilot study that you will need to conduct yourself.

B, as described above, is your boundary, the minimum margin of error that your study can tolerate. The value will be set by the researcher (you) and will be set relative to the estimated standard deviation and mean. We will now run through an example to illustrate this approach.

Let us say that you are investigating the body mass index (BMI) of the patients that attend your surgery. Fortunately there are quite a few studies that use BMI measurements so finding an estimate for the standard deviation is relatively easy. Vazquez et al. (2007) published a meta-analysis that examined the relationship between various measures of obesity and their ability to predict incipient diabetes. Across the studies they report a mean BMI of 25.8 with a standard deviation of 3.1. We will use this value of standard deviation in our example.

It is important to note that care needs to be taken when selecting a study from which to draw a standard deviation as the studied population should match that of your study as closely as possible. In the study of Vazquez et al. (2007) their populations were drawn largely from individuals attending doctors' surgeries and health clinics, and their meta-analysis also covered several countries. The mean BMI (and possibly the SD) would have been different if the population had been drawn from individuals attending an exercise gym. Sometimes of course it is not possible to get a close match between a previously published study and that of your intended study, in which case you will either have to use what you can find and accept its limitations or perform a pilot study.

The boundary value (B) must be decided by the researcher. In the context of BMI it is known that relatively small changes have little clinical significance and that BMI is not a measure of obesity that is entirely valid on its own (e.g. it tends to predict short, heavy, but lean individuals as overweight). To change BMI by one point tends to require quite a large change in body mass, thus for this example the boundary will be set at 0.5. That is, we want to know that our sample is capable of estimating the population mean to within ± 0.5 with 95 per cent confidence.

Now that all the data required to predict the required sample size are available:

$B = 0.5$

$\sigma = 3.1$

$z = 1.96$

All that is necessary is to plug the values into the equation given above:

$$\left(z_{\alpha/2} \frac{\sigma}{B}\right)^2 < n$$

Thus we have:

$$\left(1.96 * \frac{3.1}{0.5}\right)^2 < n$$

Which reduces down to:

$$(1.96 \times 6.2)^2 < n$$
$$= (12.15)^2 < n$$
$$= 147.6$$

Thus, in order to estimate the population mean to within ± 0.5 with 95 per cent confidence a minimum sample of 148 people will be required. The researcher will now be able to determine if this level of sample is within the resources available to the study. If it isn't, it may be possible to reconsider the boundary value; widening the boundary will reduce the required sample size. For example, reducing the boundary to ± 0.5 reduces the samples size to 37. If, however, this is not acceptable then the study will need to be abandoned.

Notice how we rounded up the sample required; this is because it is obviously rather difficult to sample part of a person. Thus, when quoting predicted sample size, remember to round the value to a whole number.

Predicting sample sizes for statistical test

As we said in the introduction, the power of a statistical test is in part determined by the type of statistical test being used. So, the exact nature of the power analysis will depend on the statistical test chosen. Below we look at two ways of determining samples size, one suitable for the paired t test, the other for the student's t test.

Sample size determination: one sample test

The power of a statistical test is determined by the value of $1 - \beta$ (1 – beta), where beta is the probability of a type II error. A type II error is the failure to reject a false null hypothesis. $1 - \beta$ is the probability of rejecting the null hypothesis when it is false and the alternative hypothesis is correct. In general, we want this value to be as high as possible, that is we want as much power as we can get, although Cohen (1988) suggested that a value of 80 per cent was optimum. As it is power that we are after, the method we use to predict an appropriate sample size needs to include an estimate of $1 - \beta$.

To explore this further the example described above will be used, except that this time, rather than just being interested in determining the mean BMI, we want to know if individuals that take part in a walking club show a change in BMI three months after the practices input in the clinic has ceased. You identify that this is a study that would be suitable for a paired t test (Figure 18.2). You note also that there is just one sample. The next step you may want to take is to determine the sample size that you require. The equation that you will need is as follows:

$$\frac{\left(z_{a/2} + z_{\beta-1} \right)^2 \sigma^2}{B^2} < n$$

Notice how we use the t distribution this time to determine the appropriate values for alpha and beta. As before we can read the value for alpha (the minimum significance value we wish to work at, in this example $P = 0.05$) and the value for beta from tables of the z distribution. In theory these values should be derived from the t distribution, but in practice we can only locate the t values when we know the sample size.

In this example we will set $1 - \beta$ to be 90 per cent ($P = 0.9$) and alpha to be 0.05. We will use the same value as in the previous examples (0.5) for β, the minimum margin of error, but we cannot

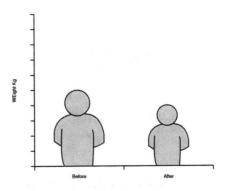

FIGURE 18.2 Depiction of part of Chae et al.'s (2012) study. Individuals' BMI was measured before and after an exercise-based intervention

use the same value for the standard deviation. This is because in the type of statistical test that will be used we would be focusing on the mean difference between the measurements before and after the intervention rather than the actual values themselves (see Chapter 12). So we need to produce an estimate for the standard deviation of the difference in BMI that occurs. Chae et al. (2012) reported a standard deviation of 1.32 for the mean change in BMI for a population of 1,947 Koreans who took part in an exercise programme. However, they also reported that the mean change was just –0.26. In other words the variation in the extent of change in BMI swamps the mean change. This is perhaps to be expected as the general experience of exercise-based interventions is that there is wide variation in the extent of the engagement of participants in the exercise for the duration of the study. We would do well therefore to set the minimum margin of error below the expected mean change, so in this case let us use 0.13 (half the expected mean change).

Plugging these values into the equation above gives:

$$\frac{(1.96+1.282)^2 * 1.32^2}{0.13^2} < n$$

which becomes:

$$\frac{18.2}{0.017} > n = 1071$$

So, with an alpha value of 5 per cent (risk of type I error), $1 - \beta$ of 90 per cent (power), a standard deviation of 1.32 and a minimum margin of error of 0.017, then a sample size of at least 1,070 will be required. Chae et al.'s (2012) study had well over this number of participants.

Sample size determination: two sample test

In most health studies where there is an intervention there will normally be at least two samples, a control group as well as the intervention group. Participants will more often than not be randomly assigned to one of these groups. Following the intervention we would then test to ascertain if any difference between the changes in BMI between the two groups was significant. In this circumstance the formula for predicting sample size becomes:

$$\frac{2\left(z_{a/2} + z_{\beta-1}\right)^2 \sigma^2}{B^2} < n$$

Using the values from the previous (one-sample) example this then gives us:

$$\frac{2(1.96+1.282)^2 * 1.32^2}{0.13^2} < n = \frac{36.4}{0.017} = 2142$$

This value for n is twice that for the one-sample test, but it must be used for each group, i.e. you would need 2142 for the intervention group and 2142 for the control group. Clearly this is quite a large number of participants; and shows the potential resource needs of working with large power and low minimum margins of error.

Box 18.1

What would be the effect on the required sample size of:

- increasing the minimum margin of error to 0.26?
- reducing power to 70 per cent?

Power analysis and statistical tests

The exact type of power analysis that you will need to do will depend on the nature of the statistical test that you wish to carry out. Power analysis software can be purchased that will estimate required sample sizes for a wide range of statistical tests. An example of such software is called PASS. PASS is able to perform power analysis for over 150 statistical tests (see www.ncss.com).

Adjust for reality

Having done a power analysis to estimate a required sample size you then need to adjust for reality. More often than not people undertaking research in the health field are working with human participants and human participants seldom behave as ideally as we would like them to. They do things such as failing to show up to appointments, moving house out of the area and not always complying with your research protocol. All this means that you generally need to adjust upwards the sample size estimates produced by power analysis. Performing a pilot study can help give you a handle on how much you may need to increase your sample.

A word on effect size

In Chapter 9 we mentioned the difference between statistically significant and 'significant implications for health care'. Just because we find a result to be statistically significant does not mean that we should act on it. Say, for example, you instigated a programme of education to help reduce the incidence of teenage (under-18) pregnancy. Your study used a large sample size and you found that the participants that received the intervention had a lower incidence of pregnancy (46/1000) than those that didn't (47/1000). Although the difference was found to be statistically significant, the difference is actually quite small.

To help decide an observed difference a measure of effect size can be calculated. Effect size is a calculation of the difference between the treatment and the control groups which standardizes the measurement of effect such that all effect sizes could be shown on a common scale. This allows different interventions to be compared.

Typically effect size is calculated by subtracting the difference of the mean result of the treatment (intervention) group from the control and dividing the resulting value by the standard deviation of the control group. Cohen (1988) developed a rule of thumb for interpreting effect size calculations. He suggested that if the result was < 0.1 the effect size was trivial; between 0.1 and 0.3 the effect was small; between 0.3 and 0.5 the effect was moderate; and > 0.5 the effect was large.

Effect size is not dependent on sample size. Prior knowledge of a particular potential effect size can help you to determine the size of sample to collect. In theory where there is a large effect size a lower sample size is required to generate a significant result. However, this argument is a bit circular, for if you know that the effect size is large, do you need to be conducting a study in the first place?

Having read this chapter and completed the exercises, you should be familiar with the following ideas and concepts:

- factors that determine the sample size that you will use;
- methods of calculating sample size;
- effect size.

EXERCISES

1. Using the standard deviation for the variable 'height' from the study on Symphadiol presented in Chapter 5, determine the sample size required to obtain a reasonable estimate of the population mean.
2. In this study you wish to perform a *t* test between group 1 and group 2 with an alpha of 0.05 and a power level of 80 per cent; estimate the sample size you will require.
3. Using the same study, calculate the effect size of the different groups. Would you introduce this drug into clinical practice? What more information would you need?

19

Analysing data from systematic reviews

Areas of learning covered in this chapter

- How can I use statistics to help inform care decisions?
- What are NNTs and L'Abbé plots?
- How are NNTs and L'Abbé plots calculated?

There are many books that look at the research process. Most of these books will provide guides to looking at the quality of published research, and we urge you to use such sources, so as to become an accomplished critical reader and user of research. The aim of this chapter is to introduce two statistical procedures that can help you look at published work and decide whether or not the procedure or practice will be of benefit to your clients or patients. The focus of this chapter will be on work that has been published in systematic reviews. The two procedures we will introduce are known as L'Abbé plots and number needed to treat (NNT).

Before we talk about these procedures we will first just note a few important points about using research from other people's studies. The first and possibly the most important principle is that of 'reader beware'; quite simply, you can't blame the author if it doesn't work for you, or if the study is poor. It is up to you to make a decision on the worth and applicability of the work to your patients or clients. You need to think about things like the sample sizes, the study populations, whether your patients are the same type of patients as those used in the study, was the study randomized, was it a **double-blind study** and does the analysis seem sensible.

The advantage of using a systematic review is that authors should clearly state what quality criteria they used for the study to be included in their review, and of course the review should contain the majority of the available studies published on a particular subject.

L'Abbé plots and NNT help us to give clinical and practical meaning to the numerical data published in clinical studies. Most of this type of data resides in the medical literature. However, as roles within the caring professions change it is important that the basis on which clinical decisions are made are understood by all health practitioners.

Number needed to treat

Box 19.1   Clinical trials

A clinical trial is where a particular intervention is put under a rigorous test. In these trials some of the participants are given the intervention, whilst other receive no treatment or a placebo. The latter group is the control.

1. Review some clinical trials; observe how the outcomes of the trials are expressed.
2. What is a placebo, and why is it used?
3. Can a placebo be an effective treatment?

If you read through some reviews or even original papers that discuss new clinical procedures you will notice that quite often the final result is given in terms of risk. In addition, the statistical analysis is often focused on whether there is a difference between the treatment and control rather than the magnitude of the difference (i.e. how well does the treatment work). Indeed this goes back to the discussion in Chapter 9 on the difference between statistical and clinical significance.

The 'risks' published are nearly always expressed in terms of a probability and therefore a value from 0 to 1 (see Chapter 10). The risk is the chance of an event, e.g. a disease, occurring. If the treatment is beneficial the risk of the event occurring should decrease in relation to the control group. For example, if you treat a group of individuals who have an open wound with an appropriate antibiotic, and another group with a placebo, the risk of infection should be less in the treatment group. It is important to remember, however, that in the case of the antibiotic treatment aimed at 'cure' rather than prevention, we would expect the number of 'events', i.e. 'cured', patients to increase in the treatment group.

The NNT statistic gives us a value that suggests how many patients we would need to treat in order to achieve the desired outcome in one individual. Ideally the NNT should therefore be 1, i.e. treat one patient and obtain one beneficial effect. In real life, however, this is seldom the case.

To illustrate we will use the following example taken from a systematic review published by Moore and Philips (1996). In their review they looked at the effectiveness of protein pump inhibitors and histamine antagonists as treatments for reflux oesophagitis, which is a condition whereby the stomach contents are regurgitated into the oesophagus. In most people this condition is rare, but in some it can become frequent and the acid nature of the stomach contents can cause considerable damage to the oesophagus. One of the studies Moore and Philips (1996) looked at involved the use of the drug Omeprazole, which is a protein pump inhibitor. We will follow their results.

In the Omeprazole review, the study group was divided into three, a control group and two experimental groups, each of which received a different dose of the drug. The experimenters found that they achieved the same outcomes irrespective of the dose and so NNT was calculated by combining both experimental groups. In total, forty-six patients were assigned to the control group and 184 to the treatment group. Of the control (placebo group) seven showed the desired outcome, i.e. recovery, whilst in the treatment group 134 did. This is all the information we need to calculate the relative and absolute risk as well as the NNT.

Box 19.2 Prophylaxis and treatment

In the case of a prophylactic intervention, it is appropriate to talk in terms of the intervention reducing the risk of the pathology occurring. In the case of treatments of an existing condition, it is less appropriate and here we talk about the risk of an event.

The risk, in this case of the treatment working for the experimental group, is 134/184 = 0.72 and in the case of the control is 7/46 = 0.15. This tells us that of 100 people on the treatment seventy-two will have a positive outcome, whilst of 100 people in the placebo group only fifteen will have a positive outcome. Any comparison of treatments will need to take into account the fact that some of the 'treatment effect' may be in fact be 'placebo' in nature. The relative event risk is the likelihood of the event, with the treatment divided by that with the placebo, 0.72/0.15 = 4.8. This suggests that a positive outcome is 4.8 times more likely with treatment than with placebo.

The only problem with relative risk is that if the control effect is small and treatment effect also small but bigger than the control the relative event risk can also be high.

The alternative if one is to present data in the form of risks is to present the absolute differences between treatments and control groups. This is known as the **absolute risk reduction** (ARR). In the case of our example this would be 0.73 − 0.15 = 0.58. This figure represents the difference in chance of the event between the two groups. It tells us how much of the overall increase in chance of a positive outcome for patients in the treatment group can be put down to the treatment. The absolute risk thus tells us more about the clinical impact of the treatment; however, it isn't easy to link directly to a clinical situation. NNT is a method that seeks to convert these risk values into a figure that practitioners can immediately relate to.

Box 19.3 Level of NNT

For treatments of existing conditions, NNTs in the order of 1–4 should be considered good. For prophylaxis, NNTs will normally be lower.

Systematic reviews tend to give the ARR provided with absolute risk reduction. The NNT is easy to calculate, as it is the reciprocal of the ARR i.e.

$$NNT = \frac{1}{ARR}$$

For our example the NNT $= \dfrac{1}{0.58} = 1.72$

This means that for every 1.72 patients treated one will show a positive outcome.

If ARR is not given then NNT can be calculated from the basic clinical trial data, i.e. the data that gives the samples sizes and outcomes from the trials. Given these data NNTs can be calculated thus:

$$NNT = \dfrac{1}{(Pos_t / Tot_t) - (Pos_c / Tot_c)}$$

Where Pos_t = Number of patients with positive outcome in treatment group

Tot_t = Total number of patients in treatment group

Pos_c = Number of patients with positive outcome in control group

Tot_c = Total number of patients in control group

In our example the values are $NNT = \dfrac{1}{(134/184) - (7/46)} = 1.72$

It is possible to compute confidence limits for NNTs. The confidence limit tells you where the 'true' population NNT lies (see Chapter 11). The calculation for confidence limits is rather complex so we have not included it in this introductory book.

Box 19.4 Positive outcome

We use the term 'positive outcome'. In a trial involving a prophylactic treatment the positive outcome will probably be no occurrence of the pathology. If you keep to this terminology there is no need to rearrange the equation to take into account different approaches to care.

NNTs can be calculated for all the studies on a particular intervention, or therapy. They can also be formulated for the range of potential treatments available. The NNTs can then be used to help select the best available option. It should not be forgotten that choice of treatment depends on a range of factors, which would include factors such as cost, patient preferences and carer experience, skill and judgement.

Example from the literature 19.1   Comparing NNTs from a range of studies

There is a wide range of analgesics available for health care professionals to use with their patients and clients. An article from the *Bandolier*, an online evidence-based journal, presents NNT data for a range of analgesics. This work allows a quick comparison to be made of the effectiveness of differing pain-relieving drugs. Take care when reading this article to note that pain relief can depend on a variety of contextual factors, such as the type of patient and their condition type. The article can be found at: www.medicine.ox.ac.uk/bandolier/booth/painpag/Acutrev/Analgesics/Leagtab.html.

We can also use the same process as outlined above to look at side effects. In this case rather than calculating a numbers needed to harm or NNH. A value can be indicated that indicates how many patients 'need' to be treated before one adverse response is observed. In general, however, one needs to search wider for reports of adverse reactions, although a good starting point is to look at the numbers of individuals withdrawn from clinical trials due to intervention related reasons.

L'Abbé plots

L'Abbé plots allow a simple graphical representation of the data from clinical trials. They involve taking the data from systematic reviews and plotting it in a way which makes it relatively easy to draw conclusions about the best available option, or at least to get a handle on the range of variation within a set of clinical trials.

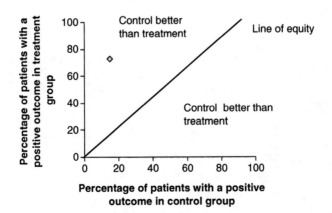

FIGURE 19.1   Modified L'Abbé plot, showing line of equity a point for a single clinical trial with the drug Omeprazole used to treat reflux oesophagitis

In a L'Abbé plot, the data from each single clinical trial form one datum point. The percentage of patients that show a positive outcome with the control form the *x*-axis and the percentage of patients that show a positive outcome with the treatment form the *y*-axis. A point is plotted were the measure for the control and treatment meet.

A line can be drawn at 45° across the graph. This represents equity, i.e. no difference between control and treatment. Trials that fall above the line of unity represent trials where benefit over and above the control treatment was shown, whilst those that fall below that line indicate that the control was better than the treatment.

We have modified the L'Abbé plot such that we show the percentage of patients with a positive outcome rather than 'those that improved with treatment' as used in the original L'Abbé plot. The use of this latter term forces the positions of the points of the graph to reverse in cases where prophylaxis is considered. The point shown on the graph is that for the example based on the use of Omeprazole that we have discussed above. When many such points are plotted it allows the level of variability within clinical trials of a specific treatment to be seen, and a consideration of its overall efficacy to be made. Similar plots for alternative treatments aid in the decision as to which treatment to adopt.

Having read this chapter and completed the exercises, you should be familiar with the following ideas and concepts:

- risk, and evaluating treatments; numbers needed to treat (NNT);
- numbers needed to harm (NNH);
- L'Abbé plots;

- how the type of intervention (prophylaxis or treatment) may influence the NNT score;
- how to use NNTs and L'Abbé plots to help determine appropriate care plans and treatments.

Find a systematic review (or several single clinical trials) of an intervention you are interested in, calculate a NNT for each study discussed in the review and produce a L'Abbé plot. (a) Do you think the intervention is effective? (b) In what circumstances is it not appropriate?

20

Choosing test statistics

Choosing the correct statistic is sometimes a hard task. The important thing to remember is to think about and decide on the statistics that you will use before you start the study. It is a good idea to write down some hypothetical data for your study and see how it fits into your proposed statistical test. The flow chart is designed to help you select an appropriate test. The chart cover statistics covered in this text. They are not exhaustive and once you make a choice make sure read about the test. This diagram applies only to the inferential statistics mentioned in this book. Do remember that this book is designed as an introduction to statistics and as such the statistics described do not represent all those available. If you design a study but cannot decide on an appropriate statistical analysis, do speak to someone knowledgeable about statistics before starting.

To choose a statistical test you must consider the scale your data have been collected on. You need to decide what phenomena you are studying, how your data are distributed and the number of groups (treatments) or sets of data that will be involved in the test. In addition, you need to consider any additional restrictions on the test, for example sample size. We have included a brief summary for descriptive statistics at the end of Chapter 6. If your studying involves using data from systematic reviews, Chapter 17 will be of use.

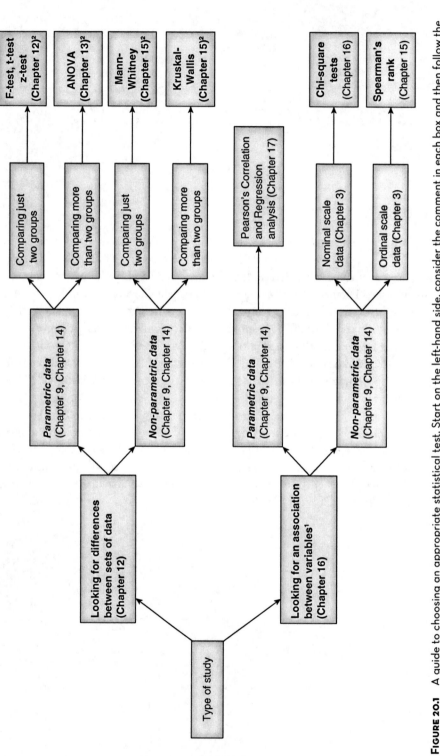

Figure 20.1 A guide to choosing an appropriate statistical test. Start on the left-hand side, consider the comment in each box and then follow the arrows to each potential decision, pick an option and follow that route. Notes: (1) It's not always immediately obvious whether you are really looking for difference or association, but if your null hypothesis can be most clearly stated using the word relationship you need a test for association. (2) The test varies depending on whether the samples are repeat measures or independent. See the chapters for detail

Appendix 1

The common symbols and abbreviations used in statistics

± plus or minus

Σ sigma, sum of (add up the values that follow)

χ Chi

μ the arithmetic mean of the population

σ (sigma) the population standard deviation

σ^2 the variance of the population

= equals

+ plus

− minus

/ divide

> greater than

< less than

π (pi) a constant of value 3.142

√ square root

P probability

s standard deviation of the sample

s^2

x̄ arithmetic mean

x a case or a value

a intercept of a straight line equation

b slope of a straight line equation

H_1 alternative hypothesis

H_o null hypothesis

CL confidence limits

d.f. degree of freedom

SD standard deviation

SE standard error

Appendix 2

A guide to critically analysing statistics

This section is intended as a guide to the critical analyses of the statistical components of research, not as a guide to overall research critique.

We suggest that you practise critically evaluating research. To do this choose some quantitative research reports on a topic that interests you and work through them, using this guide. Discuss your conclusions with your colleagues.

Population and sample

The very first thing we always look at is whether or not the sample is representative of the population. So you need to look at the size of the sample in relation to the extent of the variation in the phenomena being measured. You need to look how the sample was drawn from the population (was it random?). Look and think about biases. If information is given about how the sample was collected treat the report sceptically. If the data are normally distributed, what size are the standard errors? If these aren't given, calculate them from the standard deviation and the sample size. Always treat studies with small sample sizes with suspicion. It is unlikely the sample was representative of the wider population. Examine the researcher's attempts to analyse how close their sample was the real population of interest in detail.

Co-variables and hypotheses

Do the statistical tests applied actually test what the researchers say they want to test? A well and clearly stated hypothesis should facilitate the correct use of statistics. The most common error to look for is the use of a one-tailed instead of a two-tailed test. The other most frequent mistake is failure to take into account a co-variable or extraneous variables. A similar problem can also stem from design when subjects are not truly randomly distributed amongst treatment groups (again likely to be a problem with small data sets) or if groups have not been matched properly (again likely to be a problem with small data sets).

Data description and presentation

Have appropriate summaries of the data been provided, including measures of central tendency and dispersion (Chapter 6)? Do the types of measure provided match the type of data recorded? Are the data clearly presented using suitable tables, graphs and figures (Chapter 7)? What do the descriptions tell you about the data? Can you get a feel for what the data looks like? For example, how can you tell how the data are distributed?

Choice of statistical analysis

Does the choice of statistical test suit the data under investigation? Is the test suitable for:

- number of treatments or groups;
- the number of variables;
- and the measurement scale(s) used to collect the data.

Has a justification been made for the choice of statistical test? If parametric tests have been used have the authors tested to see if the data examined do not deviate from the normal distribution (Chapter 9)? If non-parametric alternatives have been used are they suitable? Have the appropriate corrections been made (Chapter 14)?

Check that the numbers add up, for example that the appropriate number of degrees of freedom has been used and that the outcome of the statistical tests seems to tally with the description of the data.

Are the statistical tests appropriate to the hypothesis being tested? If a one-tailed test is used is it justified?

Discussion

Has the correct hypothesis been rejected/accepted? Are the statistics integrated into the discussion and used with due caution and regard to the determined statistical significance level? Do the researchers keep their discussion within the boundaries of their sample and population? It is quite common for researchers to extrapolate their findings beyond the original population. If the null-hypothesis is not rejected be suspicious of any reasons that are put forward to suggest why the hypothesis was not confirmed. A perfectly well-designed study should not allow room for justification as to why the hypothesis may still hold true if it was rejected. We have to acknowledge that we do not live in a perfect world, but nevertheless reasons should be well justified and not anticipated before the onset of the study.

Appendix 3

Statistical tables

TABLE 1 Percentage points of the F distribution, v1 = degrees of freedom of sample with larger variance and v2 the degrees of freedom of the sample with the smaller variance 0.05 level of significance

v1	1	2	3	4	5	6	7	8	9	10	12	24	120	infinity
v2														
1	161.4	199.5	215.7	224.6	230.2	234.0	236.8	238.9	240.5	241.9	243.9	249.1	253.3	254.3
2	18.51	19.00	19.16	19.25	19.30	19.33	19.35	19.37	19.38	19.40	19.41	19.45	19.49	19.5
3	10.13	9.55	9.28	9.12	9.01	8.94	8.89	8.85	8.81	8.79	8.74	8.64	8.55	8.53
4	7.71	6.94	6.59	6.39	6.26	6.16	6.09	6.04	6.00	5.96	5.91	5.77	5.66	5.63
5	6.61	5.79	5.41	5.19	5.05	4.95	4.88	4.82	4.77	4.74	4.68	4.53	4.40	4.36
6	5.99	5.14	4.76	4.53	4.39	4.28	4.21	4.15	4.10	4.06	4.00	3.84	3.70	3.67
7	5.59	4.74	4.35	4.12	3.97	3.87	3.79	3.73	3.68	3.64	3.57	3.41	3.27	3.23
8	5.32	4.46	4.07	3.84	3.69	3.58	3.50	3.44	3.39	3.35	3.28	3.12	2.97	2.93
9	5.12	4.26	3.86	3.63	3.48	3.37	3.29	3.23	3.18	3.14	3.07	2.90	2.75	2.71
10	4.96	4.10	3.71	3.48	3.33	3.22	3.14	3.07	3.02	2.98	2.91	2.74	2.58	2.54
11	4.84	3.98	3.59	3.36	3.20	3.09	3.01	2.95	2.90	2.85	2.79	2.61	2.45	2.40

(Continued)

TABLE 1 (Continued)

v1 v2	1	2	3	4	5	6	7	8	9	10	12	24	120	infinity
12	4.75	3.89	3.49	3.26	3.11	3.00	2.91	2.85	2.80	2.75	2.69	2.51	2.34	2.30
13	4.67	3.81	3.41	3.18	3.03	2.92	2.83	2.77	2.71	2.67	2.60	2.42	2.25	2.21
14	4.60	3.74	3.34	3.11	2.96	2.85	2.76	2.70	2.65	2.6	2.53	2.35	2.18	2.13
15	4.54	3.68	3.29	3.06	2.90	2.79	2.71	2.64	2.59	2.54	2.48	2.29	2.11	2.07
16	4.49	3.63	3.24	3.01	2.85	2.74	2.66	2.59	2.54	2.49	2.42	2.24	2.06	2.01
17	4.45	3.59	3.20	2.96	2.81	2.70	2.61	2.55	2.49	2.45	2.38	2.19	2.01	1.96
18	4.41	3.55	3.16	2.93	2.77	2.66	2.58	2.51	2.46	2.41	2.34	2.15	1.97	1.92
19	4.38	3.52	3.13	2.90	2.74	2.63	2.54	2.48	2.42	2.38	2.31	2.11	1.93	1.88
20	4.35	3.49	3.10	2.87	2.71	2.60	2.51	2.45	2.39	2.35	2.28	2.08	1.90	1.84
21	4.32	3.47	3.07	2.84	2.68	2.57	2.49	2.42	2.37	2.32	2.25	2.05	1.87	1.81
22	4.30	3.44	3.05	2.82	2.66	2.55	2.46	2.40	2.34	2.30	2.23	2.03	1.84	1.78
23	4.28	3.42	3.03	2.80	2.64	2.53	2.44	2.37	2.32	2.27	2.20	2.01	1.81	1.76
24	4.26	3.40	3.01	2.78	2.62	2.51	2.42	2.36	2.30	2.25	2.18	1.98	1.79	1.73
25	4.24	3.39	2.99	2.76	2.60	2.49	2.40	2.34	2.28	2.24	2.16	1.96	1.79	1.71
26	4.23	3.37	2.98	2.74	2.59	2.47	2.39	2.32	2.27	2.22	2.15	1.95	1.75	1.69
27	4.21	3.35	2.96	2.73	2.57	2.46	2.37	2.31	2.25	2.20	2.13	1.93	1.73	1.67
28	4.2	3.34	2.95	2.71	2.56	2.45	2.36	2.29	2.24	2.19	2.12	1.91	1.71	1.65
29	4.18	3.33	2.93	2.70	2.55	2.43	2.35	2.28	2.22	2.18	2.1	1.9	1.70	1.64
30	4.17	3.32	2.92	2.69	2.53	2.42	2.33	2.27	2.21	2.16	2.09	1.89	1.68	1.62
40	4.08	3.23	2.84	2.61	2.45	2.34	2.25	2.18	2.12	2.08	2.00	1.79	1.58	1.51
60	4.00	3.15	2.76	2.53	2.37	2.25	2.17	2.10	2.04	1.99	1.92	1.7	1.47	1.39
120	3.92	3.07	2.68	2.45	2.29	2.17	2.09	2.02	1.96	1.91	1.83	1.61	1.35	1.25
infinity	3.84	3.00	2.60	2.37	2.21	2.10	2.01	1.94	1.88	1.83	1.75	1.52	1.22	1.00

TABLE 2 Percentage points of the *F* distribution, v1 = degrees of freedom of sample with larger variance and v2 the degrees of freedom of the sample with the smaller variance 0.01 level of significance

v1	1	2	3	4	5	6	7	8	9	10	12	24	120	infinity
v2														
1	4052	4999.5	5403	5625	5764	5859	5928	5982	6022	6056	6106	6235	6339	6366
2	98.5	99.00	99.17	99.25	99.30	99.33	99.36	99.37	99.39	99.40	99.42	99.46	99.49	99.5
3	34.12	30.82	29.46	28.71	28.24	27.91	27.67	27.49	27.35	27.23	27.05	26.6	26.22	26.13
4	21.2	18	16.69	15.98	15.52	15.21	14.98	14.8	14.66	14.55	14.37	13.93	13.56	13.46
5	16.26	13.27	12.06	11.39	10.97	10.67	10.46	10.29	10.16	10.05	9.89	9.47	9.11	9.02
6	13.75	10.92	9.78	9.15	8.75	8.47	8.26	8.1	7.98	7.87	7.72	7.31	6.97	6.88
7	12.25	9.55	8.45	7.85	7.46	7.19	6.99	6.840	6.72	6.62	6.47	6.07	5.74	5.65
8	11.26	8.65	7.59	7.01	6.63	6.37	6.18	6.03	5.91	5.81	5.67	5.28	4.95	4.86
9	10.56	8.02	6.99	6.42	6.06	5.8	5.61	5.47	5.35	5.26	5.11	4.73	4.40	4.31
10	10.04	7.56	6.55	5.99	5.64	5.39	5.2	5.06	4.94	4.85	4.71	4.33	4.00	3.91
11	9.65	7.21	6.22	5.67	5.32	5.07	4.89	4.74	4.63	4.54	4.40	4.02	3.69	3.6
12	9.33	6.93	5.95	5.41	5.06	4.82	4.64	4.5	4.39	4.30	4.16	3.78	3.45	3.36
13	9.07	6.7	5.74	5.21	4.86	4.62	4.44	4.3	4.19	4.10	3.96	3.59	3.25	3.17
14	8.86	6.51	5.56	5.04	4.69	4.46	4.28	4.14	4.03	3.94	3.8	3.43	3.09	3.00
15	8.68	6.36	5.42	4.89	4.56	4.32	4.14	4.00	3.89	3.80	3.67	3.29	2.96	2.87
16	8.53	6.23	5.29	4.77	4.44	4.2	4.03	3.89	3.78	3.69	3.55	3.18	2.84	2.75
17	8.4	6.11	5.18	4.67	4.34	4.10	3.93	3.79	3.68	3.59	3.46	3.08	2.75	2.65
18	8.29	6.01	5.09	4.58	4.25	4.01	3.84	3.71	3.6	3.51	3.37	3.00	2.66	2.57
19	8.18	5.93	5.01	4.50	4.17	3.94	3.77	3.63	3.52	3.43	3.30	2.92	2.58	2.49
20	8.1	5.85	4.94	4.43	4.1	3.87	3.7	3.56	3.46	3.37	3.23	2.86	2.52	2.42
21	8.02	5.78	4.87	4.37	4.04	3.81	3.64	3.51	3.4	3.31	3.17	2.80	2.46	2.36

(Continued)

TABLE 2 (Continued)

v1	1	2	3	4	5	6	7	8	9	10	12	24	120	infinity
v2														
22	7.95	5.72	4.82	4.31	3.99	3.76	3.59	3.45	3.35	3.26	3.12	2.75	2.40	2.31
23	7.88	5.68	4.76	4.26	3.94	3.71	3.54	3.41	3.3	3.21	3.07	2.70	2.35	2.26
24	7.82	5.61	4.72	4.22	3.9	3.67	3.5	3.36	3.26	3.17	3.03	2.66	2.31	2.21
25	7.77	5.57	4.68	4.18	3.85	3.63	3.46	3.32	3.22	3.13	2.99	2.62	2.27	2.17
26	7.72	5.53	4.64	4.14	3.82	3.59	3.42	3.29	3.18	3.09	2.96	2.58	2.23	2.13
27	7.68	5.49	4.6	4.11	3.78	3.56	3.39	3.26	3.15	3.06	2.93	2.55	2.2	2.1
28	7.64	5.45	4.57	4.07	3.75	3.53	3.36	3.23	3.12	3.03	2.90	2.52	2.17	2.06
29	7.6	5.42	4.54	4.04	3.73	3.5	3.33	3.2	3.09	3.00	2.87	2.49	2.14	2.03
30	7.56	5.39	4.51	4.02	3.7	3.47	3.3	3.17	3.07	2.98	2.84	2.47	2.11	2.01
40	7.31	5.18	4.31	3.83	3.51	3.29	3.12	2.99	2.89	2.8	2.66	2.29	1.92	1.8
60	7.08	4.98	4.13	3.65	3.34	3.12	2.95	2.82	2.72	2.63	2.50	2.12	1.73	1.6
120	6.85	4.79	3.95	3.48	3.17	2.96	2.79	2.66	2.56	2.47	2.34	1.95	1.53	1.38
infinity	6.63	4.61	3.78	3.32	3.02	2.80	2.64	2.51	2.41	2.32	2.18	1.79	1.32	1

TABLE 3   *t* distribution

Significance	0.05	0.01	0.001
d.f.			
1	12.71	63.66	636.62
2	4.30	9.92	31.60
3	3.18	5.84	12.92
4	2.77	4.60	8.61
5	2.57	4.03	6.87
6	2.45	3.71	5.96
7	2.36	3.50	5.41
8	2.31	3.35	5.04
9	2.26	3.25	4.78
10	2.23	3.17	4.59
11	2.20	3.11	4.44
12	2.18	3.06	4.32
13	2.16	3.01	4.22
14	2.14	2.98	4.14
15	2.13	2.95	4.07
16	2.12	2.92	4.02
17	2.11	2.90	3.96
18	2.10	2.88	3.92
20	2.09	2.84	3.85
22	2.07	2.82	3.8
26	2.06	2.78	3.7
28	2.05	2.76	3.67
30	2.04	2.75	3.64
40	2.02	2.7	3.55
60	2.00	2.66	3.46
120	1.98	2.62	3.73
infinity	1.96	2.58	3.29

Significance levels are for two-tailed tests, for one-tailed test divide significance level by two

TABLE 4   Chi-square (χ^2) distribution

d.f.	Significance Level	
	$P = 0.05$	$P = 0.01$
1	3.84	6.63
2	5.99	9.21
3	7.81	11.34
4	9.49	13.28
5	11.07	15.09
6	12.59	16.81
7	14.07	18.48
8	15.51	20.09
9	16.92	21.67
10	18.31	23.21
11	19.68	24.72
12	21.03	26.22
13	22.36	27.69
14	23.68	29.14
15	25.00	30.58
16	26.30	32.00
17	27.59	33.41
18	28.87	34.81
19	30.14	36.19
20	31.41	37.57
25	37.65	44.31
30	43.77	50.89
40	55.76	63.69
50	67.50	76.15
60	79.08	88.38
80	101.88	112.33
100	124.34	135.81

TABLE 5　Correlation coefficients (*r*) for one-tailed test (double the significance level for two-tailed test)

d.f.	Significance Level	
	P = 0.05	*P* = 0.01
3	0.805	0.934
4	0.729	0.882
5	0.669	0.833
6	0.621	0.789
7	0.582	0.750
8	0.549	0.716
9	0.521	0.685
10	0.497	0.658
11	0.476	0.634
12	0.457	0.612
13	0.441	0.592
14	0.426	0.574
15	0.412	0.558
16	0.400	0.542
17	0.389	0.528
18	0.378	0.515
19	0.369	0.503
20	0.360	0.492
25	0.323	0.445
30	0.296	0.409
40	0.257	0.358
50	0.231	0.322
60	0.211	0.295
80	0.183	0.256
100	0.163	0.230

TABLE 6 Mann-Whitney U test values, $P = 0.05$

n_1 \ n_2	2	3	4	5	6	7	8	9	10	11	12	13	14	15	16	17	18	19	20
2							0	0	0	0	1	1	1	1	1	2	2	2	2
3				0	1	1	2	2	3	3	4	4	5	5	6	6	7	7	8
4			0	1	2	3	4	4	5	6	7	8	9	10	11	11	12	13	13
5		0	1	2	3	5	6	7	8	9	11	12	13	14	15	17	18	19	20
6		1	2	3	5	6	8	10	11	13	14	16	17	19	21	22	24	25	27
7		1	3	5	6	8	10	12	14	16	18	20	22	24	26	28	30	32	34
8	0	2	4	6	8	10	13	15	17	19	22	24	26	29	31	34	36	38	41
9	0	2	4	7	10	12	15	17	20	23	26	28	31	34	37	39	42	45	48
10	0	3	5	8	11	14	17	20	23	26	29	33	36	39	42	45	48	52	55
11	0	3	6	9	13	16	19	23	26	30	33	37	40	44	47	51	55	58	62
12	1	4	7	11	14	18	22	26	29	33	37	41	45	49	53	57	61	65	69
13	1	4	8	12	16	20	24	28	33	37	41	45	50	54	59	63	67	72	76
14	1	5	9	13	17	22	26	31	36	40	45	50	55	59	64	67	74	78	83
15	1	5	10	14	19	24	29	34	39	44	49	54	59	64	70	75	80	85	90
16	1	6	11	15	21	26	31	37	42	47	53	59	64	70	75	81	86	92	98
17	2	6	11	17	22	28	34	39	45	51	57	63	67	75	81	87	93	99	105
18	2	7	12	18	24	30	36	42	48	55	61	67	74	80	86	93	99	106	112
19	2	7	13	19	25	32	38	45	52	58	65	72	78	85	92	99	106	113	119
20	2	8	13	20	27	34	41	48	55	62	69	76	83	90	98	105	112	119	127

Values are for two-tailed test. n_1 and n_2 are the number of cases in each sample

TABLE 7 Critical values for *T* for the Wilcoxon's test for matched pairs

n	Significance Level		
	P = 0.05	*P* = 0.025	*P* = 0.01
5	$T \leq 0$		
6	2	0	
7	3	2	0
8	5	3	1
9	8	5	3
10	10	8	5
11	13	10	7
12	17	13	9
13	21	17	12
14	25	21	15
15	30	25	19
16	35	29	23
17	41	34	27
18	47	40	32
19	53	46	37
20	60	52	43
21	67	58	49
22	75	65	55
23	83	73	62
24	91	81	69
25	100	89	76
26	110	98	84
27	119	107	92
28	130	116	101

One tailed; double values for two-tailed test

Appendix 4

Answers to exercises

In this appendix we provide the answers to some of the questions provided at the end of each of the chapters. We have given definitive answers to those questions where there is a definitive answer to give. For the other questions we have suggested approaches or things to consider. In places we have also provided a comment to help you understand what we have done to find the answer. We encourage you to practise your statistics by reviewing papers, joining in research and undertaking research of your own.

Chapter 1

We are often asked to change our practice by others, and because we tend to work in hierarchical organizations we do not always consider the evidence base. Thankfully the idea of using an evidence base has now become firmly established, particularly where new or evolving health care is concerned. The questions at the end of the chapter ask you both to consider changes that you have deliberately made to your practice and those that you have been asked to make. Ask yourself questions such as what type of data was used and how it was presented. If, for example, you are following guidance on particular procedures, what type of evidence has been used to produce that guidance?

Chapter 2

In this edition we have included URLs to several open access research papers and so, as long as you have internet access, you should have no problem finding suitable papers. The questions we ask at the end of this chapter are relatively difficult because they ask you to locate the use of a particular philosophy, yet that philosophy is often not explicitly stated, but assumed. The chapter outlines certain aspects of the quantitative paradigm and with careful reading it should be possible to see some of these in action. For example, where authors use a questionnaire there is often an assumption that the phenomenon in question can be accurately and reliably measured using this questionnaire. Whilst many of the papers that we cite are seeking to establish causal links, i.e cause and effect, few discuss the notion of trying to establish 'universal laws'.

In answering the first question you will probably find that most papers do not contain an explicit discussion of each of the steps we describe as the scientific method. For example, in many articles it is relatively infrequent to find the hypothesis actually stated as such; it is more normal for it to be assumed. Similarly, the conceptual and theoretical frameworks are seldom explicitly discussed in quantitative papers.

The final question in this chapter asks you about your feelings; this is because the way we feel about evidence influences the likelihood that we will believe and act on it. Some people are much more cautious and suspicious of numerical data.

Chapter 3

In question 1 we ask you to identify the key variables within two different types of study: the sampling unit, the sample and the statistical population. In the first type of study a physical phenomenon is being studied and how it is influenced by exercise. The physical phenomenon is bone density and so this is the variable of interest. This study concerns itself with how the bone density of individual women changes over time, therefore the sample unit is individual women. The sample comprises those women who were selected and agreed to take part, whilst the statistical population comprises those who were available to be selected. It is likely that the study would make inferences to the whole population of women within this age group.

The second study is slightly different because we are interested in the occurrence of something (meningitis) within populations defined by geographic area. We are interested in this phenomenon at the level of the village and so the sample unit is 'village'. The sample would comprise those villages included in the study, whilst the study may attempt to infer its findings to all villages in south-west England. It is, nevertheless, constrained by the fact that it is possible there may be no data for some villages. An added complication in a study such as this is that the researchers would need to define quite clearly what constituted a village.

1. (i) (a) Bone density. (b) An individual woman. (c) Women aged between 35–45 who were selected and agreed to take part in the study. (d) Women aged between 35–45 who were available to take part in the study.
   (ii) (a) Incidence of meningitis. (b) Villages. (c) Villages selected for the study. (d) Villages in the south-west of England for which data are available.

Question 2 again asks you to consider the relationship between what the population could be and what in reality it was. Reconciling these two different populations and recognizing that they are different is an important aspect of research analysis. The difference between these populations can limit the extent to which research is generalizable.

2. (a) Those individuals that could potentially visit the walk-in clinic. (b) Those individuals that visit the clinic and elect to fill in the questionnaire.

In question 3, recognizing the measurement scale of different variables is important because scale type dictates the type of statistical reporting and the type of statistical analysis that can be used. In a questionnaire-type survey, often it is the researcher when designing the questionnaire who determines the scale type.

3. Age: interval. Sex: nominal. Number of partners: ordinal. Sexual activity: ordinal. Ethnic group: nominal. Barrier choice: nominal. Reason not to use barrier: nominal. Presentation: nominal.

Question 4: Sampling is a compromise. Ideally we would measure the whole population, but we seldom have the time to do this so we must sample. Very often the sample does not quite match the population. The degree of mis-match is the error that can be said to be due to the sampling. Sampling error can be defined as the difference between the parameters of the sample and those of the population.

Chapter 4

The questions asked at the end of this chapter do not have definitive answers. The first question asks you to decide which if any of the questions are leading. This is a difficult question to answer because to some extent whether or not a person is led is dependent on their personality. An aspect of question 1 that could be leading would be the order in which the various options are presented.

Question 2 focuses on reliability and validity. We ask you to decide if in the studies you select a questionnaire was the most appropriate tool. Your answer will depend on whether or not you think that the questionnaire really reflects the phenomena under research. In good studies, the researcher will rigorously explore the validity of their questionnaire and its reliability. If they do not do this, treat their results with caution.

Chapter 5

No questions.

Chapter 6

1   Mean = 2.45, Median = 1.0, Mode = 1.0.

- Median and possibly the mode. These data are not symmetrical, which dictates that you should not quote the mean as the only measure of central tendency. As these data are not nominal ordinal the median is the most suitable.
- These results suggest that the data are skewed. The mean is higher than both the mode and the median and so the data are skewed.

2   Mean = 13.53, Median = 13.50, Mode = 10 and 18 (note these data are multi-modal).

- The mean is the most appropriate, but you would probably want to signal that these data are multi-modal, i.e. that there is more than one mode.
- Multi-modal data tend to suggest that the data set represents samples from two different populations. In the case of these data this is not surprising as you have combined the data from a control and a treatment group.

3 For exercise 1, quartiles are 1.0, 1.0 and 2.0 respectively for lower, mid and upper quartiles. Standard deviation is 3.70. For question 2, quartiles are 7.25, 13.5 and 20.0 respectively for lower, mid and upper quartiles. Standard deviation is 8.0.

For exercise 2, the standard deviation is much greater than the inter-quartile ranges. The quartiles are very close together indicating data that are heavily skewed. In this case we would have quoted both the quartiles, but also the range. For exercise 2 we would have quoted the standard deviation.

Chapter 7

1. These data are most appropriate to display using a frequency bar chart, with each symptom being given a bar and the height of the bar indicating the frequency. Alternatively a pie chart could be used that displays the proportion of each symptom but also indicates the frequency.
2. These data are probably best displayed using a bar chart, with a bar for the control and one for the treatment group. The height of the bar should correspond to the mean value for each group of participants, the standard deviation could be indicated by using 'error' bars. An alternative form of presentation would be to use box and whisker plots.
3. In this exercise you are creating a time series of the change in your pulse rate over time. The most appropriate form of representation for these data would be to use a line graph, with time after you did the exercise on the x-axis and pulse rate on the y-axis. Each point (your pulse rate at a certain time) can be joined with a line, indicating that there is a link (you) between each datum points.
4. There is no definitive answer to this question.

Chapter 8

No questions.

Chapter 9

1. (a) That a daily does of Symphadiol enhances weight loss in clinically obese individuals (males, aged 30–40), compared to just using a calorie-controlled diet. (b) Symphadiol significantly increases weight loss over the course of the research in clinically obese males (aged 30–40)

on a calorie-restricted diet compared to a control group who use a calorie-controlled diet alone. (c) There is no difference in weight loss over the course of the study in clinically obese males (aged 30–40) on a calorie-restricted diet compared to a control group who use a calorie controlled diet alone. (d) Weight loss. (e) Treatment group.

2. The likely sources of error are: sampling error, the difference between the sample and the true population; variation in the sampling error between the treatment groups: measurement error, i.e. accuracy of measurement tools; accuracy of measurement recorders; design error, e.g. how was the level of compliance of the participants with the experimental design maintained; influence of confounding variables, e.g. height.

Chapter 10

1. The distribution of the data within your sample will depend on the people that you have samples of. If you have sampled both men and women it is likely that the distribution of your data will be bimodal. Conversely if you have just sampled from one gender it is more likely that the sample will be bimodal.

2. As you increase the size of the sample, the distribution will start to resemble that of the 'population'. This is because you will be reducing your sampling error. If your sample is mixed gender, as males tend to have larger hands than females, then the frequency distribution will still remain bimodal.

3. (a) H = Heads T = Tails: HHHH, TTTT, HTHH, HHTH, HHHT, HHTT, HTTT, HTHT, THTT, TTHT, TTTH, TTHH, THHH, THTH. (b) There are fourteen different combinations. It is a certainty that you will draw at least one of these combinations. Each combination has an equal chance of being drawn, therefore the probability of obtaining any one of these outcomes is 1/14 or $P = 0.0714$. (c) The probability of obtaining one tail and three heads is 0.2856. How is this? A combination that give us one tail and three heads occurs several times – THHH, HTHH, HHTH and HHHT – four times in fact, given that the probability of drawing any one of these combinations is 0.0714 (see answer to 3b). Then the probability of drawing one tail and three heads is 4 x 0.0714 or 0.2856. (d) No definitive answer.

Chapter 11

1. Mean = 179 SD = 12.25 SE = 3.16 95 per cent CI = 179 ± 6.2.

2. The standard deviation is a descriptive statistic. It tells us, assuming that the population is normally distributed, that approximately 66 per cent of the individuals in the study sample will have values for the measure within the range of the mean, plus or minus one standard deviation. The standard error (SE) is a predictive statistic. It predicts with approximately 66 per cent confidence that the population mean is with the range of the sample mean plus or minus 1 SE. The 95 per cent confidence limits extends the confidence of this prediction to 95 per cent. It is the mean plus or minus 1.96 standard errors.

3. The answer to the first two items of this question we leave to your judgement and understanding of people's behaviour. The third part illustrates how the use of statistics can help avoid situations of shortage arising or at least enable us to take a risk with a knowledge of how likely an event is to occur.

Using the z distribution it is possible to make a prediction of how many needles would be required to avoid running out. In this case you needs to find the z score in the table for the relevant percentages (in this case 65 per cent and 95 per cent) and then use the equation $z = \dfrac{x - \bar{x}}{s}$ to determine the value of x (number of needles required). In this question you would have values for the mean, standard deviation and z, so you need to rearrange the equation and solve for x. An example of this type of calculation can be found on page 165.

(i) 109 (for 95 per cent)
(ii) 88 (for 65 per ent)

Chapter 12

3, 4, 5 F test and student's t test should be performed. This is because the measurement scale is of ratio and the data are probably parametric or at least not significantly different from the normal distribution. We are looking to see whether a difference between two groups is significant and so a t test is relevant. The two groups are not connected and so an independent t test is the most appropriate form of t test. We use an F test to check for equality of variance.

The F test tells us that there is no significant difference between the variance of the two samples $F = 0.51$, $P < 0.05$ d.f. = 28. The difference between the control and the treatment group means is also not significant $t = 0.43$ $P > 0.05$ d.f. = 28 (one-tailed tests). We can conclude that there is no significant difference between the control and treatment group means.

6 Test results from education assessments tend to approximate to interval scales, although this is not always the case, so would need exploring. Assuming that the data are not significantly different from normally distributed then a t test is appropriate. This is because we are looking for a difference between the means of two groups. Clearly the participants before and after the event are the same and we are making a repeat measure on the same individual separated by an intervention. Thus a paired t test is appropriate.

There is a small (two-point) difference before and after the lectures. Paired t test (two-tailed) indicates that the difference is significant. $t = 3.83$ $P < 0.01$ d.f. = 10.

Chapter 13

5 There is no significant difference between any of the treatment groups (ANOVA $F_{3, 56} = 2.39$ $P > 0.05$). Below the ANOVA table is displayed (we preferred using a computer package because it saves time and the method does not have the added risk of arithmetic errors):

	Sum of squares	d.f.	Mean square	F	Sig.
Between groups	428.133	3	142.711	2.388	.079
Within groups	3346.800	56	59.764		
Total	3774.933	59			

We can conclude from this test that there is no significant difference between the different treatment groups or the control. The one-way ANOVA test is suitable because we want to establish whether there is a significant difference between more than two groups and these data are measured on an interval scale.

Chapter 14

1. A chi-square goodness of fit test suggests that the variable age is not significantly different from that predicted by the equation for a normal distribution. $\chi^2 = 31.36$ d.f. $= 38$ $P > 0.05$.
2. The variable number of partners has a clumped distribution. Most people have just one partner; a few people have multiple partners. You may be able to transform these data to a normal distribution using a $Log(x + 1)$ transformation.

Chapter 15

1. There is no significant difference between Asian and African participants with respect to the numbers of sexual partners recorded ($U = 29.00$ $n = 18$ $P > 0.05$). A Mann–Whitney U test has been used.
2. There is no significant difference between ethnic groups in relation to the numbers of sexual partners reported ($\chi^2 = 1.93$ d.f. $= 2$ $n = 18$ $P > 0.05$). A Kruskal–Wallis test was used in this example.
3. There is a significant negative correlation between the numbers of partners reported and the age of the participant ($r_s = -27$ $n = 40$ $P < 0.05$). Spearman's rank correlation was used to answer this question.

Chapter 16

1. There is no significant difference between the frequencies of the different presentations. However, if those presentations indicative of sexually transmitted disease are combined then the difference is significant ($\chi^2 = 12.25$ d.f. $= 10$ $P < 0.05$). The greatest difference between observed and expected values stems from the large number of presentations indicative of STDs.
2. There is no significant difference between the ethnic groups with respect to attendance at the clinic ($\chi^2 = 14.75$ d.f. $= 8$ $P < 0.05$).

Chapter 17

1. There is a significant negative correlation between weight loss and height of the participant ($R = 0.27$, $R^2 = 0.075$ $P < 0.05$). (b) The relationship is weak as the R^2 is low, just 7.5 per cent of the variation in weight loss is explained by the height of the participant; clearly there are other factors at work. (e) The slope of the regression line is weight loss (kg) = $-22.47 + 0.0202$ x height (cm). To predict the weight loss of an individual who is 170 cm tall you must put this value into the equation. The answer is 11.86 kg.

Glossary

Absolute risk   The actual probability that an event will occur.

Absolute risk reduction   The difference in the chance of an event between the treatment and control groups.

ANOVA   Stands for analysis of variance, a technique for looking for differences between means from two or more samples.

Average   A parameter that describes the central tendency of a population.

Bar chart   A graph drawn using rectangular bars to show how large each value is, the top of the bar signifies the value of interest.

Binomial distribution   A probability distribution based on the occurrence of a particular outcome based on n independent yes/no events.

Case   A single value or item of data.

Central limit theorem   The theory which predicts that the frequency distribution of the means of samples drawn from any population will approach the normal distribution.

Chance   An expression of how likely an event is to occur.

Chi-square   A statistic commonly used to compare frequencies amongst nominal level data.

Confidence limits   An expression of the range of values between which the population mean is believed to be found.

Confounding variable   A variable that hides the influence of the variable of interest, such that it is difficult to analyse.

Contingency tables   Tables that display frequency data for nominal scale data.

Continuous variable   A variable measured on the interval or ratio scales.

Control group   The participants or objects in a study to which no treatment is applied.

Correlation   A technique to look for association between variables that have been measured on either the interval, ratio or ordinal scales.

Cronbach alpha reliability coefficient   A measure of the internal consistency of a questionnaire.

Degree of freedom   A number used in statistical calculations based on the sample size and used because we are working on samples not whole populations.

Dependent variable   The values of this variable are dependent on those of another.

Double-blind study   A study where neither the participants nor the researchers know who is in the control and treatment groups.

Experimental group   The participants or objects in a study to which a treatment is applied.

Extraneous variable   A variable that has not been controlled for or measured

***F* test for equality of variance**   A statistical test to determine the likelihood that the variances between two samples are significantly different.

Face validity   Refers to whether or not the content of a questionnaire reflects the subject matter.

Frequency distribution   A graphical representation of the numbers of times each potential value actually occurs in a sample.

Goodness of fit   A statistical test to help evaluate how well an ideal mathematical frequency distribution fits the observed distribution.

Histogram   A graphical display of frequencies where the data are grouped into ranges.

Hypothesis   The proposition or prediction that is being tested when using statistics.

Independent variable   The values of this variable are thought to influence the value of other variables (dependent variables) in the study.

Interval/ratio scale   Types of measurement scale where the distance between the points of the scale are mathematically the same and quantified in absolute terms.

Kruskal–Walis test   A non-parametric equivalent of the one-way ANOVA.

Kurtosis   One of the measures of the shape (flatness) of frequency distributions.

L'Abbé plot   A method of plotting the results from clinical trials.

Linear regression   A statistical technique for describing the linear relationship between two variables that are thought to be related.

Mean   A measure of central tendency, the sum of all the values divided by the number of values.

Measurement   The establishment of a parameter of a person or object.

Measurement error   The error that is made when measuring the value of a variable phenomenon.

Median   The geometric mean; the physical middle value when all the values are lined up in numerical order.

Metrics   A quantitative measurement.

Mode   The most common value in a series of values or cases.

Nominal scale   A scale of measurement where data are assigned to a category that is given a name; the data cannot be put into a sequence.

Non-parametric test   Statistical test which does not rely on the data being distributed in a manner that approximates to a defined mathematical distribution.

Normal distribution   A frequency distribution where the mean, median and mode are identical and the mean ± standard deviation encloses 68.26 per cent of all the cases.

Number needed to treat   The numbers of individuals that you need to treat before being able to measure a positive benefit to one individual.

Null hypothesis   The opposite of the hypothesis being tested, normally that there is no difference between the means or frequencies from different samples.

One-tailed test   A test where the hypothesized difference is predicted to be in one direction from the mean.

Ordinal scale   A scale of measurement where the values imply an order although the magnitude of the difference between values on the scale is not known.

***P*value**   The numerical expression of probability ranges from 1.0 = certainty to 0.0 = impossible. Often quoted to indicate significance or otherwise.

Paired *t* test   A technique for establishing differences between means of two related samples.

Paradigm   A way of thinking shared by a majority.

Parameter   The measures which describe the variables of a sample.

Parametric tests   Statistical tests that make the assumption that the data are distributed approximately according to a defined mathematical distribution.

Percentage   A proportion multiplied by 100.

Placebo   An object or activity that is almost identical to the experimental treatment accepted that it has no or very limited biological activity, often used to provide the control treatment in clinical trials.

Poisson distribution   A type of frequency distribution that describes events that occur rarely.

Population   All the individuals or objects that meet your studies requirements and that you could potentially gather information from.

Power   The probability of rejecting the null hypothesis when it should be rejected.

Power analysis   A technique to help determine the likelihood of a statistical test refuting the null hypothesis.

Probability   An expression of how likely an event is to occur, expressed as a number where $1.0 =$ certain and $0.0 =$ impossible.

Proportion   Ratio of the number of one category of cases in relation to the total number of cases.

Qualitative data   Data which are concerned with describing meaning which is normally word based.

Quantitative paradigm   A world-view that phenomena can be quantified and measured, predicted and variation controlled for.

Quartile   The physical values at the points that divide the data into quarters when all the values are lined up in numerical order.

Questionnaire   A research tool that uses a series of questions to elicit responses from the participants.

Random   An event or pattern in which all outcomes are equally likely.

Random sample   Each member of the population has an equal chance of being selected.

Regular distribution   A distribution where the standard deviation is small relative to the mean.

Reliability co-efficient   A measure of the reliability of a research tool.

Repeat measures design   Tests that investigate difference between samples, where the samples are made of the same individuals.

Representativeness   Refers to how closely what is being measured is to what the researcher actually wants to investigate.

Robust   Refers to statistical tests, which if some of their assumptions are broken nevertheless retain their power.

Sample   A subset of the population.

Sampling error   The difference between the parameters of the population and those of the sample.

Sampling unit   Persons or object that individual measurements are taken from.

Significance   A statement that suggests the observation being examined is unlikely to have occurred by chance and therefore should be considered 'real' should be accompanied by a statement rejecting the null hypothesis and with the level of significance (P value).

Skew   A measure of how symmetrical a frequency distribution is.

Standard deviation   A measure of the level of deviation from the mean expressed in a standardized form.

Standard error   A measure of the difference between the sample mean and the population mean.

Statistically significant   Where a statistical test infers that a result has not occurred by chance.

Student's *t* test   A technique for establishing differences between means of two independent samples.

Survey   A research method designed to gather information about a population that can be descriptive comparative or attitudinal.

Systematic error   Error caused by any factors that systematically affect measurement of the variable across the sample. For example, a thermometer that tended not to measure accurately across the whole range of temperatures under study would introduce a systematic error. This type of error is also called *bias*.

Target group   The individuals within a population that a researcher is interested in sampling from.

Transformation   A technique to change the mathematical form of data so that it is more easily analysed.

Treatment group   The participants or objects in a study to which the experimental procedure is applied.

Two-tailed test   A test were the hypothesized difference from the mean does not have a specified direction.

Type I error   Rejecting the null hypothesis when it is true.

Type II error   Not rejecting the null hypothesis when it should be rejected.

Variable   A phenomenon or thing that relates to the individual or objects under study that varies.

Variance   A measure of how much variation there is in a set of data.

Wilcoxon's test   A non-parametric test that is similar to the paired *t* test.

z score   A measure of how many standard deviations an individual case is from the mean.

References

Acklin, M.W and Bernat, E. (1987) Depression, alexithymia, and pain prone disorder: a Rorschach study. *Journal of Personality Assessment* 51(3): 462–79.

Allison, P.D. (1999) *Multiple Regression*. London, Sage Publications

Balcázar, H., Alvarado, M., Hollen, M.L., Yanira, G.-C. and Pedregón, V. (2005) Evaluation of Salud Para Su Corazón (Health for Your Heart) – National Council of La Raza Promotora Outreach Program. *Preventing Chronic Disease* 2(3): A09.

Bandolier (2007) Oxford league table of analgesics in acute pain. www.medicine.ox.ac.uk/bandolier/booth/painpag/Acutrev/Analgesics/Leagtab.html.

Bannister, C., Ballards, C., Lanna, M., Fairbairn, A. and Wilcock, G. (1998) Placement of dementia sufferers in residential and nursing home care. *Age and Ageing* 27: 189–93.

Bates, D.M. and Watts, D.G. (1988) *Nonlinear Regression Analysis and Its Application*. New York, Wiley.

Blaikie, N. (2003) *Analysing Quantitative Data*. London, Sage.

Burns, R. (2000) *Introduction to Research Methods* (4th rev. edn). London, Sage.

Caplan, G.A., Meller, A., Squires, B., Chan, S. and Willett, W. (2006) Advance care planning and hospital in the nursing home. *Age and Ageing* 35(6): 581–5.

Castle, N. (2004) Family satisfaction with nursing facility care. *Journal for Quality in Health Care* 16(6): 483–9.

Chae, J.S., Kang, R., Kwak, J.H., Paik, J.K., Kim, O.Y., Kim, M., Park, J.W., Jeon, J.Y. and Lee, J.H. (2012) Supervised Exercise Program, BMI, and Risk of Type 2 Diabetes in Subjects with Normal or Impaired Fasting Glucose. *Diabetes Care* 35(8): 1680–5.

Chen, J.L.-Y., Cheng, J. C-H., Kuo, S.-H., Chan, H-M., Huang, Y.S. and Chen, Y.-H. (2013) Prone breast forward intensity-modulated radiotherapy for Asian women with early left breast cancer: factors for cardiac sparing and clinical outcomes. *Journal of Radiation Research* 1–10. doi: 10.1093/jrr/rrt019.

Chung, S-C., Gedeborg, R., Owen, N., James, S., Jeppsson, A., Wolfe, C., Heuschmann, P., Wallentin, L., Deanfield, J., Timmis, A., Jernberg, T., and Hemingway. H. (2014) Acute myocardial infarction: a comparison of short-term survival in national outcome registries in Sweden and the UK. *The Lancet* 23 January (DOI: 10.1016/S0140-6736(13)62070-X).

Cohen, J. (1988) *Statistical Power Analysis for the Behavioral Sciences* (2nd edn). Hillsdale, NJ: Lawrence Erlbaum.

Collison, D., Dey, C., Hannah, G. and Stevenson, L. (2007) Income inequality and child mortality in wealthy nations. *Journal of Public Health* 29 (2): 114–17.

Colyer, H. and Kamath, P. 1999 Evidence-based practice. A philosophical and political analysis: some matters for consideration by professional practitioners. *Journal of Advanced Nursing* 29(1): 188–93.

Depoy, E. and Gitlin, L.N. (1993) *Introduction to Research*. St Louis, MO, Mosby.

Gage, W., Heywood, S. and Norton, C. (2012) Measuring quality in nursing and midwifery practice. *Nursing Standard* 26(45): 35–40.

Gibbs, G. (2010) *Dimensions of Quality*. York, Higher Education Academy.

Gillham, B. (2008) *Developing a Questionnaire (Real World Research)*. London, Continuum International.

Goldacre, B. (2013) Are clinical trial data shared sufficiently today? No. *British Medical Journal* 347:f1880.

Griffiths, P., Harris, R., Richardson, G., Hallett, N., Heard, S. and Wilson-Barnett, J. (2001) Substitution of a nursing-led inpatient unit for acute services: randomized controlled trial of outcomes and cost of nursing led intermediate care. *Age and Ageing* 30(6): 483–8.

HMRC (2005) www.hmrc.gov.uk/stats/income_distribution/table3-2-2004-05.pdf.

Huff, D. (1973) *How to Lie with Statistics*. London, Penguin Books.

Kalisch, J., Tschannen, D. and Kyung, L. (2011) Do staffing levels predict missed nursing care? *International Journal for Quality in Health Care* 23(3): 302–8.

Kerr, A.W., Hall, H.K. and Kozub, S.A. (2002) *Doing Statistics with SPSS*. London, Sage Publications.

Kjeldsen, S.E., Hedner, T., Jamerson, K., Julius, S., William, E.H., Zabalgoitia, M., Butt, A.R., Rahman, S.N. and Hansson, L. (1998) Hypertension optimal treatment (HOT) study, home blood pressure in treated hypertensive subjects. *Hypertension* 31: 1014–1020. Available at http://hyper.ahajournals.org/content/31/4/1014.full.

Maben, J., Morrow, E., Ball, J., Robert, G. and Griffiths, P. (2012) *High Quality Care Metrics for Nursing*. London, National Nursing Research Unit, King's College London.

Marsh, P. and Kendrick, D. (1998) Injury prevention training: is it effective health education research? *Theory & Practice* 13(1): 47–56.

Maynard, A. (2003) 'Tribes in need of data?' Business and management, *The Times Higher Education Supplement*, May, p. 26.

Moore, R.A. and Philips, C. (1996) Reflux Oesophagitis; quantificative systematic review of the evidence if the evidence of the effectiveness of protein pump inhibitors and histamine antagonist. http://ebandolier.com/bandopubs/gordf/gord.html.

The NHS Information Centre, Prescribing and Primary Care Services (2010) *Quality and Outcomes Framework: Achievement Data 2009/10*. The Health and Social Care Information Centre. Available at: https://catalogue.ic.nhs.uk/publications/primary-care/qof/qual-outc-fram-09-10/qof-09-10-rep.pdf (accessed 15 October 2013).

NHS Outcomes Framework 2012/2013. London, Department of Health.

North West Transparency Project UK (2012) www.bfwh.nhs.uk/toc_mar2012.pdf (accessed 2 May 2012).

Office for National Statistics (2011) *Mortality Statistics: Deaths Registered in England and Wales (Series DR) - 2010*. www. ons.gov.uk/ons/index.html.

Oppenheim A.N. (1992) *Questionnaire Design, Interviewing and Attitude Measurement*. London. Pinter.

Pittet, D., Hugonnet, S., Harbath, S., Mourouga, P., Sauvan, V., Touveneau, S. and Perneger, T.V. (2000) Effectiveness of a hospital-wide programme to improve compliance with and hygiene. *The Lancet*, October, 356: 307–312.

Popper, K. (1959) *The Logic of Scientific Discovery*. London, Hutchinson.

Raleigh, V. and Foot, C. (2010) *Getting the Measure of Quality*. London, King's Fund.

Royal College of Nursing (RCN) (2009) *Measuring for Quality in Health and Social Care: An RCN Position Statement*. London, Royal College of Nursing.

Royal College of Nursing (RCN) (2011) *Nursing Dashboards – Measuring Quality*. London, Royal College of Nursing.

Sandqvist, G., Scheja, A. and Hesselstrand, R. (2010) Pain, fatigue and hand function closely correlated to work ability and employment status in systemic sclerosis. doi:10.1093/rheumatology/keq145.

Shickle, D., Hapgood, R. and Qureshi, N. (2002) The genetics liaison nurse role as a means of educating and supporting primary care professionals. *Family Practice* 19(2): 193–6.

Sivenius, J., Pyörälä, K., Heinonen, J.O., Salonen, P.T. and Riekkinen, P. (1985) The significance of intensity of rehabilitation of stroke – a controlled trial. *Stroke* 16: 928–93.

Sokal, R.R. and F. J. Rohlf. (2012) *Biometry: The Principles and Practice of Statistics in Biological Research*, 4th edition. New York: W. H. Freeman and Co.

UKCC (1983) *Nursing Research: The Role of the UKCC*. London, UKCC.

Vazquez, G., Duval, S., Jacobs, Jr., D.R. and Silventoinen, K. (2007) Comparison of body mass index, waist circumference, and waist/hip ratio in predicting incident diabetes: a meta-analysis. *Epidemiologic Reviews* 29(1): 115–28.

Wang, T. and Palese, P. (2009) Unravelling the mystery of swine influenza virus. *Cell* 137(6): 983–5.

Zebiene, E., Razgauskas, E., Basys, V., Baubiniene, A., Gurevicius, R., Padaiga, Z. and Svab, I. (2004) Meeting patients' expectations in primary care consultations in Lithuania. *International Journal of Quality Health Care* 16(1): 83–9.

Index

CPSIA information can be obtained at www.ICGtesting.com
Printed in the USA
LVOW09s1803131215

466483LV00007B/151/P

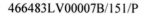